KETO·GENESIS

30 WELL FED DAYS TO A NEW, LEANER & HEALTHIER YOU

ALICIA TOBIN, R.H.N. & CHRIS GURSCHE

FORESIGHT PUBLISHING

This book may be ordered from **www.ketogenesis.ca**

Published by Foresight Publishing
New Westminster, BC

Printed in Canada
Friesens Corporation, 2015

Cover and Book Design by Andrea Schmidt (a-schmidt.com)
Photography by Matt O'Donnell
Food Styling by Alyssa Robertson, R.H.N.

ISBN 978-0-9940637-0-0
www.ketogenesis.ca
First edition

Library and Archives Canada Cataloguing in Publication

Tobin, Alicia, author
      Keto·Genesis / Alicia Tobin, R.H.N. and Chris Gursche.

Includes index.
ISBN 978-0-9940637-0-0 (BOUND)

      1. Ketogenic diet. 2. Cookbooks. I. Gursche, Chris,
author II. Title.

RC374.K46T62 2015   641.5'631   C2015-901356-9

CONTENTS

FOREWORD

AS A NATUROPATHIC DOCTOR I spend a large portion of my time evaluating the individual terrain of the body. With a focus on integrative oncology, I look at factors that may have caused cancer and other chronic diseases. I also evaluate and consider the obstacles that potentially stand in the way of successful treatment. The old saying "you are what you eat" still holds true to this day. The western diet has caused an epidemic of insulin resistance and an overindulgence of sugar, carbs and disease-feeding foods. We live in a sugar addicted society and subsequently are seeing a higher incidence of cancer, obesity, fatigue and chronic diseases. Although the cause of this is beyond multi-factorial, the one thing we do have great control over is our diet and lifestyle. We know that we can exercise more, stress less, sleep longer and try our best to stay away from toxins. However, we live in a constantly changing society where science and medicine make new claims each day and it becomes increasingly difficult to decide which diet to follow.

If you are reading this you have most likely done some research on the ketogenic diet and have even glanced through these wonderful recipes and ideas by Alicia Tobin and Chris Gursche. I have successfully treated patients using different variations of the ketogenic diet. These patients range from weight loss, neurological disease or injury, chronically ill and of course, cancer.

In my experience the diet can be extremely challenging without the proper training and planning. This cookbook is a great tool for those wanting to start the diet, providing access to delicious healthy coaching in the form of recipes. It is hard not to be healthy when the food tastes this good! Many of my patients notice weight loss, gains in athletic performance, more consistent energy, shifts to their glucose and insulin pathways, visible improvements to their skin and – most importantly – positive changes to their state and prognosis of chronic disease. According to the research, each individual generally has to eat a specific amount of carbohydrates daily, based on their diagnosis and goals. The wonderful thing about this book is the layout of net carbohydrates. The reader can navigate through their daily diet based on how many carbohydrates they are allowed to consume. The higher carbohydrate recipes are extremely easy to substitute without affecting taste. As you shift into ketosis while enjoying these meals, recognize that you have taken a major step into treatment and prevention of illness. If you have been using the ketogenic diet for some time, enjoy the new flavours this cookbook provides. Throughout your journey, take the time to thank yourself for committing to a healthier you.

– *Dr. Janelle Murphy B.Sc. (kin), N.D.*

ACKNOWLEDGMENTS

SINCERE THANKS TO CHRIS GURSCHE

for the opportunity to write a cookbook, certainly a chance I would never have turned down, and to Karla for opening up your home for photo shoots. Matt O'Donnell and Alyssa Robertson for being the best and bravest for taking on the photos and food styling, and Andrea Schmidt for being a life-long friend. Everyone at Alpha Health Products for tasting and testing recipes. And a hearty thank you to Marianne Robertson for helping not only with editing, but also for being an amazing sous chef. My mother Leah, and my dad Michael, I love you very much. And to my friends who are like family. And if you bought this book – thank you too! xoxo

– Alicia Tobin, R.H.N.

BESIDES THE PEOPLE ALICIA HAS THANKED,

I need to thank Alicia. This project would not have happened without her, and I couldn't have asked for a better partner. Matt and Alyssa played big roles keeping everyone on track, and if the food looks good, you have them to thank. And Ovi, who is rarely out front, for keeping all the numbers straight.

I also need to acknowledge, and am grateful for, the assistance from my lovely wife Karla, my daughters Katrina and Korinna, my mother Christel, and Matt's wife, Melissa, who all willingly pitched in on the big photo shoot days, playing the roles of chefs, sous chefs, and dishwashers. And of course my sister Silke, who came to the rescue with two breakfast recipes when my mind was all but numb.

I am surrounded by willing, able, talented people, and my life is richer for it. I trust that our combined efforts will make your life richer as well. Bon Appétit.

– Chris Gursche

PREFACE

THIS BOOK IS INTENDED to be used as a food plan for people who follow a ketogenic lifestyle. A ketogenic diet is one in which fat, from good quality sources, accounts for the highest calorie intake, carbohydrates the lowest, while low to moderate amounts of protein are consumed. This triggers a process in the body known as nutritional ketosis, where fat becomes the primary energy source, not carbohydrates. It can be especially beneficial for people who have trouble losing weight or must restrict carbohydrates to support a specific condition.

We have written 30 days' worth of recipes to mix and match that are nutritious and, as importantly, delicious. We hope that these meals inspire you to try new takes on favourite meals so your goals of better health are supported while you feel nourished inside and out. The recipes have a net carb count (total carbs minus fibre equals net carbs) and a protein count to help you choose something just right for your mood and daily carb count. Our recipes are almost all gluten-free, and many can be made vegetarian or even vegan to fit the needs of the reader or a special dinner guest. Please look for our handy carb and protein counts and the occasional recipe tip to help you eat some pretty great meals.

Chris and I were inspired by our own thoughtful and ardent pursuit of finding foods and meals that keep us happy and healthy. We also want our readers to be active participants in their wellness and to be curious about how our diets play a key role in our health. Simply put, when you eat well, you start to feel well.

Collaborating on a cookbook also brought together two very different points of view, palates, and political views, and I am grateful to Chris not only for the opportunity to write with him but also as a Holistic Nutritionist to have grown to understand why everything must be braised. Hopefully Chris understands why I rant about quality ingredients and pastured meats.

We have had many laughs and late nights of cooking, and now, this wonderful book to share with you.

– Alicia Tobin, R.H.N.

METRIC CONVERSION CHART

IN THIS COOKBOOK we have followed the metric system to provide accurate measurements for the total carbohydrate and protein conversions, which is important when following a ketogenic diet. For your ease and reference, below are simple conversion charts you can refer to.

SOLIDS, FRESH HERBS & CARBOHYDRATE-HEAVY ITEMS

FOOD CATEGORY	METRIC MEASUREMENT	IMPERIAL EQUIVALENT
Vegetables, shredded or fine dice	100g	1 cup
Vegetables, chopped	150g	1 cup
Fruits, chopped	125g	1 cup
Avocado, large	200g	1 cup
Garlic cloves	3–4g	1 clove
Fresh lighter herbs (e.g., cilantro, dill)	40g	1 cup
	3g	1 tablespoon
Fresh heavier herbs (e.g., basil, rosemary)	75g	1 cup
	5g	1 tablespoon
Light greens, chopped (e.g., spinach, lettuce)	30–40g	1 cup
Heavy greens, chopped (e.g., kale, chard)	65g	1 cup
Flour	120g	1 cup
	5g	1 tablespoon
Coconut Sugar	160g	1 cup
	6g	1 tablespoon
Flaxseed	10g	1 tablespoon
Hemp hearts	10g	1 tablespoon
Pecans and Walnuts	100g	1 cup
Almonds	150g	1 cup
Cheese, grated	100–120g	1 cup

LIQUIDS, DRIED HERBS & SPICES

METRIC MEASUREMENT	IMPERIAL EQUIVALENT
1.25 mL	¼ teaspoon
2.5 mL	½ teaspoon
5 mL	1 teaspoon
15 mL	1 tablespoon
60 mL	¼ cup
80 mL	⅓ cup
125 mL	½ cup
250 mL	1 cup
1L	4 cups

Please note: these are approximate conversions, and will not always be exact. These are based on our measurements for items used regularly throughout the cookbook.

A NOTE ON INGREDIENTS

BOTH CHRIS AND I AGREE that the best ingredients make eating well a better experience. In our cookbook we have made note of particular products we enjoy using, and believe to be the best available on the market. If an ingredient or brand is not available to you locally, ask at your market or health food store what they would recommend. This also opens up the opportunity to try new combinations and to make the recipe your own.

Fats and the quality of the oil you use in preparation and for cooking require special consideration. We use a variety of safe fats for cooking: coconut oil, red palm oil and olein, butter, camelina oil and ghee. These oils are safe for cooking. Animal fats may be used as well, but we don't prefer them.Sometimes we call for sautéing in Alpha Balance™ Oil. This should only be done on low heat. Please do not use any other oils for cooking.* In some cold or room temperature recipes we used high quality organic, unfiltered extra virgin olive oil.

In many cases we used full fat organic yogurt instead of mayonnaise, it works well and is very low in carbs. All of the salad dressings are using good quality oils, fresh herbs, and are simple to make. The sugars we used, if any, are minimally refined: honey, maple syrup, and coconut blossom sugar.

We invite you to start switching to organic produce, nuts, grains and seeds. Get familiar with either your local farmer or farmers market where you can really see where your food comes from. Sustainably sourced fish, and the animals that are not factory farmed but have access to a better quality of life. Please source grass-fed and pastured dairy, beef, lamb and pork. When buying products sourced from the developing world, we buy fair trade wherever possible.

We like quality organic yogurt and kefir, we love Saugeen Country brand. Butter made from grass-fed dairy cattle is best and your organic grocer will have at least one option for you. For soy sauce alternatives we like gluten-free tamari, coconut aminos, and especially Bragg's.

Alpha Health Products sponsored some of our kitchen ingredients. Alpha sources and manufactures premium oils: award-winning fair trade virgin organic DME™ Coconut Oil (our ethical and flavour favourite), Alpha Organic Camelina Oil, Alpha Organic Fair Trade Red Palm Olein (sustainably sourced), Alpha Balance™ (now organic), Organic Coconut Blossom Sugar, and Organic Coconut Flour. These products are available for purchase at **www.alphahealth.ca** or at your local health food store. Thank you so much for your support!

Baking is a different matter. Oils that cannot withstand cooking heat may be used in baking because of the dispersion of the oil through the food, as well as the protection of being within the baked goods. Our favourites here are still coconut oil, red palm fruit shortening, and butter, although Alpha's Energy™, Balance™, and Clarity™ oils may be used to increase the ketogenic values.

HOW TO BE WELL FED

WHEN I LOOK AT THE RISE of chronic illness, obesity, and the epidemic of type 2 diabetes in North America, I always feel frustrated because what our bodies require to be healthy, and how they function, is largely ignored or misunderstood. We are told by refined food manufacturers that their products are healthy and safe, but what we aren't told is that most of those products aren't really food at all. The food that the vast majority of people eat is refined, and really no longer a food, but a product formulated to be cheap and addictive and to leave the body wanting more. We are not well fed people. We are starving for nutrients.

Sadly, we are not taught how to eat, nor how to grow, and certainly not to cherish food or those who produce it for us. When I see a body that is overweight, I really see a person who is starving for good food. Real food. There are so many healthy body types, and your goal shouldn't be to be thin. It should be to be well fed. Our relationship with food is a very deep and important one and it takes time. But our bodies respond quickly and favourably when we start eating real food. Our bodies know what they need to work, we just have to start listening to them.

How can you be well fed? The solution is to eat a diet of nutrient-dense foods, drink adequate water, and if you aren't already doing so, to begin exercising. These three things could change your whole relationship with your body. No one can do this for you but yourself, and you are going to need to start trusting that your body will respond to eating real food. It is what we were meant to do all along. Your relationship with food is one of the most important relationships you have, because what you eat has a direct impact on who you are and how you feel.

I want to be well fed and I want you to be too. I encourage you to begin listening to your body. When you crave sweets, eat fruit. When you want a burger, make one. If you are an adult who hates vegetables, grow up. Know where your food comes from. Go to the farmers market and buy fresh, gorgeously imperfect produce, real eggs, and meat from animals that had happy lives.

Be well fed.

— Alicia Tobin R.H.N

KETO·GENESIS: LEAN, HEALTHY & FULL OF ENERGY

THE STORY OF THIS BOOK begins with my father Siegfried Gursche. Together with Dr. Mary Newport, he worked out a formula for an oil blend that had beneficial effects on people with Alzheimer's, stopping their memory degradation, and lifting the mental fog. Mary's husband Steve had been diagnosed with a case of early onset. Through Dr. Newport's connection with Dr. Richard Veech, they came to understand that the operational principle behind the oil blend was ketones.

The trick, however, is in elucidating exactly how ketones work. That's where I come in. I'm one of those people who needs to figure out how stuff works. I can't tell you the number of appliances that I've disassembled in my past that have never made it back together again. This need set me on a journey that not only answered how ketones are effective for people with neurodegenerative diseases like Alzheimer's, Parkinson's, ALS, glaucoma, and quite potentially, MS, but also how ketones are effective for people like me, who just want to be lean and healthy. And full of energy.

I believe it's important to understand how ketones are made in the first place. Ketones are a result of fat metabolism in the liver. This happens when there are a high level of free fatty acids, created in the first step of fat metabolism circulating in your bloodstream.

The liver scavenges approximately 30% of free fatty acids from the bloodstream, and starts to catabolize them, that is, break them down through a process called beta-oxidation. The final product of this catabolism is a two carbon unit molecule with a co-enzyme tail called acetyl-coenzymeA. When there are a lot of these molecules present at one time, they tend to acidify the environment. To bring the body back to homeostasis, a place of neutrality, two of these molecules are hooked together into a ketone body or what we refer to as ketones. Ketogenesis, then, is the formation of ketone bodies through the metabolic utilization (catabolism) of fats.

Ketones are wonderful little energy units because they are water soluble, meaning they can be freely carried around to the various cells via the bloodstream. Ketones can cross the blood brain barrier, meaning they can nourish the brain as well. One of the real benefits of ketones over glucose, the fuel made from breaking down carbohydrates, is that ketones do not require insulin to get into the cells. That makes ketones extremely effective in cases of insulin deficiency, as happens in diabetes, or glucose uptake impairment, which is one of the issues with brain cells in Alzheimer's. Ketones also lead to a higher level of energy production than can be made from glucose. Research indicates that ketones are actually the body's preferred source of fuel. That makes sense when you consider that in pre-agricultural societies, carbohydrates would have been difficult to come by.

Let's talk about carbohydrates for a second. Carbohydrates, or carbs, have become the predominant fuel in our culture. We've all heard of simple carbs and complex carbs. Eventually they all break down into glucose that our bodies use as fuel. The problem is that an excess of glucose is toxic, so the body must clear it from the bloodstream. It does this by releasing insulin, which opens up glucose gates in the cells, removing the glucose from the blood. The glucose that is not required for energy in the cells is turned into fat for storage.

Should the body undergo a period of glucose deprivation, the body releases the stored fats as fatty acids into the bloodstream. When these fatty acids reach the liver, they are converted into ketones to be used for energy. The reason why this doesn't happen all the time is that the presence of insulin stops the process of ketone production, since insulin in the blood is a signal that the body has more than enough energy available. The process is a metabolic brake to make sure that precious energy isn't wasted. This is a great mechanism when the chance of you eating dinner depends on whether the sabre-tooth tiger stops circling the tree you're sitting in. When you live in a society where the slightest hunger pang can be filled with a 2000 calorie meal within seconds of having responded to "May I take your order, please," the results are an excess of stored energy, particularly around the middle.

The upshot is that the average well fed person, consuming about 70% of their energy intake in the form of carbohydrates, has less than 1mg of ketones circulating per deciliter of blood. That measurement translates to less than .1mmol for those scoring on home blood ketone meters. The indications are that a glucose fed metabolism, reliant upon insulin, is more prone to chronic inflammatory degenerative diseases. This is not yet established science, but there sure are a lot of fingers pointing that way.

The purpose of this book is to show you the way to breaking the reliance on glucose as your primary fuel, switching over to good fats for a leaner, healthier outcome. There are a few things that you need to know to be successful.

First, there is a conversion table. We have made our recipes in grams and millilitres not because we are hard core Canadian metric users, but because gram weights are more accurate than ounces, and weights are more accurate than volume measurements. How many carbohydrates are there in a half cup of pineapple? That depends on whether you're talking tidbits, or chunks, or really big chunks, the way I like to eat pineapple. But 50g of pineapple is the same, no matter how it's cut.

The measurements are there in case you have a requirement for strictness in your eating. This would be because you are using diet as a treatment for a degenerative disease (hopefully in conjunction with your health care provider), or because you wish to lose several inches in waist measurement quickly. The other reason we measure is to provide you with a frame of reference as to how many carbs and proteins you can expect from any given food. If your goal is to find your natural lean, and get there on your own time, then the measurements are less critical.

In the scientific literature, there is a range of what is considered a ketogenic diet. Some, like Dr. Thomas Seyfried of Boston University, have used diets restricted to 20 net grams of carbs per day, and limited protein, to successfully shrink cancer tumors. Dr. Peter Attia recommends between 30 to 50 carbs per day. Our position is that 50g of net carbohydrates, and moderated protein, will move you into a state of ketogenesis, and keep the insulin levels within the range of normal resting states, even after eating a meal. Again, unless you have particular therapeutic requirements, that's a sustainable and satisfactory place to be.

It is important for us that this be a way of eating, rather than a diet. There are no restrictions in ketogenic eating, other than staying within the carbohydrate limits and moderating the protein intake. You can achieve ketogenesis as a vegetarian, a vegan (though this is difficult and will require planning), under a gluten-free diet, or even as dairy-free.

Ketogenesis is different than Paleo and Atkins, primarily in that we recommend the limitation of the daily intake of protein to 1g per kg of bodyweight. Even that is on the high side, and it is suggested we don't need more than .65g / kg to fuel our bodily processes. If you ingest more protein than your body requires, the excess is turned first into glucose, potentially triggering an insulin response, and then into body fat. That is one reason why you may not lose fat on an Atkins diet plan. We also recommend that if you eat meat, you eat all the cuts, not just the lean. There are several braises in this book, which are an excellent way of making use of the cheaper cuts. Soooo tasty.

Finally, if you've picked up this book because your primary goal is to drop inches off your waistline, I've got good news for you. The process works. One of the benefits of eating low carb, moderated protein, fat to satiation is the satiation part. You don't leave the table hungry, which is the best way to ensure you stick with a plan. The other benefit is that fats carry the flavours in food, and all the herbs and spices don't have any carbs to speak of. Typically, all the herbs and spices in our meals add up to less than 1 net gram of carbs. That is one well spent carb. So the food is flavourful and filling – what's not to like?

Sometimes people have a bit of trouble getting ketogenesis going in their bodies. When I started, I was measuring my ketones and was sure my meter was broken, since the needle never moved. Then I went to a picnic and got food poisoning. Two days of not eating and suddenly my liver was generating ketones. I'm not suggesting you get food poisoning, but a one or two day fast might be a good way to start off.

If you have a need to lose fat more quickly, say to get a metabolic issue under control, then you may combine ketogenic eating with calorie restriction to good effect. Intermittent fasting or the 5-2 plan definitely work. I tried the 5-2 plan for about 3 months. My mantra on the restricted calorie days was "tomorrow, I can eat anything I want." As I look back on it now, on those restricted calorie days, I was eating ketogenically, only without the "fat to satiation" part. So I added fat. I'm still slimming down, although slowly.

Our hope in presenting this information is that you will find tasty recipes that please your palate and satisfy you, body and soul. But also that you will take these as a starting point, to learn what it is to eat ketogenically, and adapt and rework to suit your lifestyle and your nutritional and taste requirements. As we say in our house, "Guten Appetit," which my non-German friends have degraded to "Good enough to eat." And so it is.

Happy Keto·Genesis.

– *Chris Gursche*

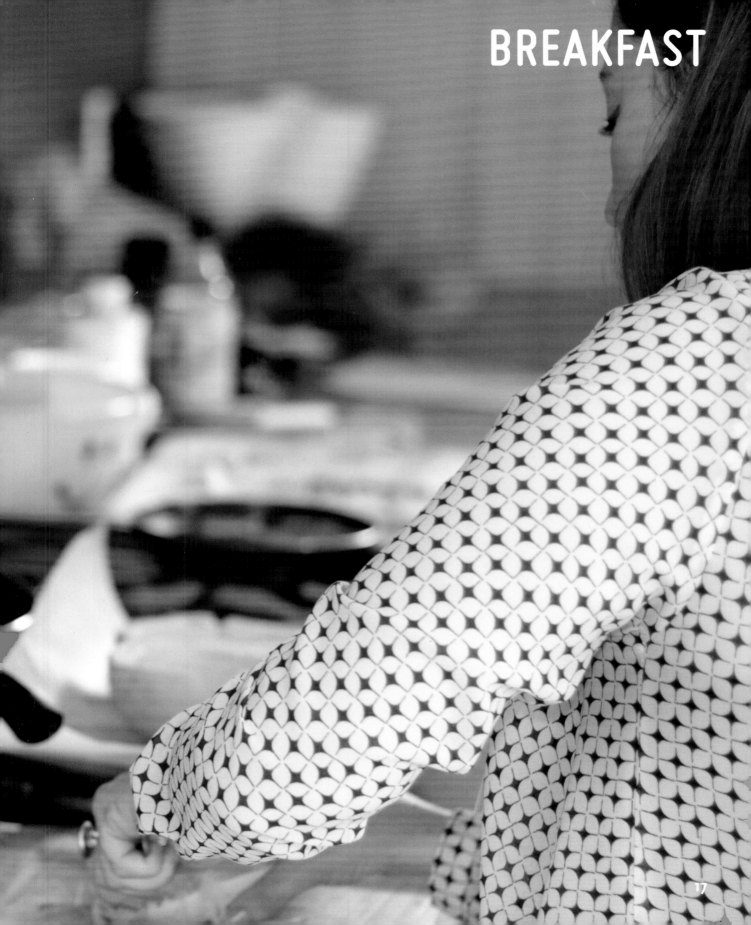

APPLE BREAKFAST MUFFINS

Makes 24 muffins | Ready in 30 minutes

200g almonds, ground
5g flaxseed, fresh ground
1 mL salt
2 mL baking soda
1 egg
125 mL milk
15 mL melted butter
250g (2 small) Granny Smith apples,
    peeled and cored

No added sugar! These mini muffins are great for a quick grab-and-go breakfast. Combine them with an Alpha Energizer Coffee (recipe follows) for a perfect start to your day. —CG

PREHEAT oven to 175°C (350°F).

COMBINE the dry ingredients in a small bowl. In a medium bowl, whisk the eggs, then add the milk and butter, and whisk thoroughly to combine. Gradually whisk the dry ingredients into the egg mixture.

LINE mini-muffin tin with paper liners. Scoop about 15 mL into each liner. Bake for 20 minutes.

NET CARBS 2.1G	PROTEIN 2.3G PER MUFFIN

GF   VEG

ALPHA ENERGIZER COFFEE

Makes 1 cup | Ready in 5 minutes

250 mL brewed coffee or espresso
15 mL DME™ Coconut Oil
15 mL butter

BLEND and enjoy!

NET CARBS 0G	PROTEIN .1G PER SERVING

GF   VEG

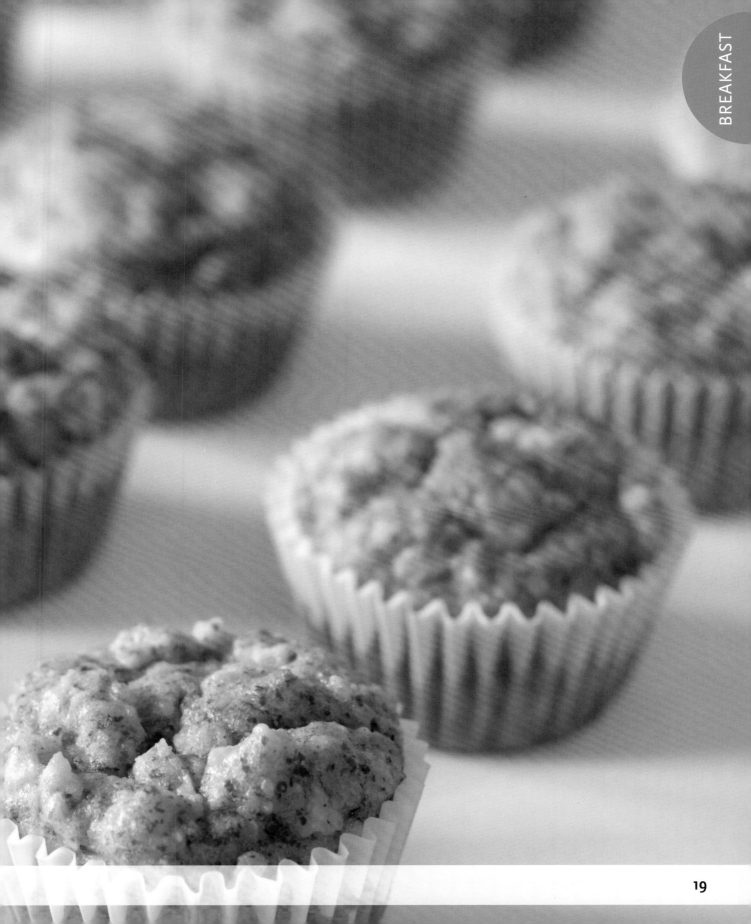

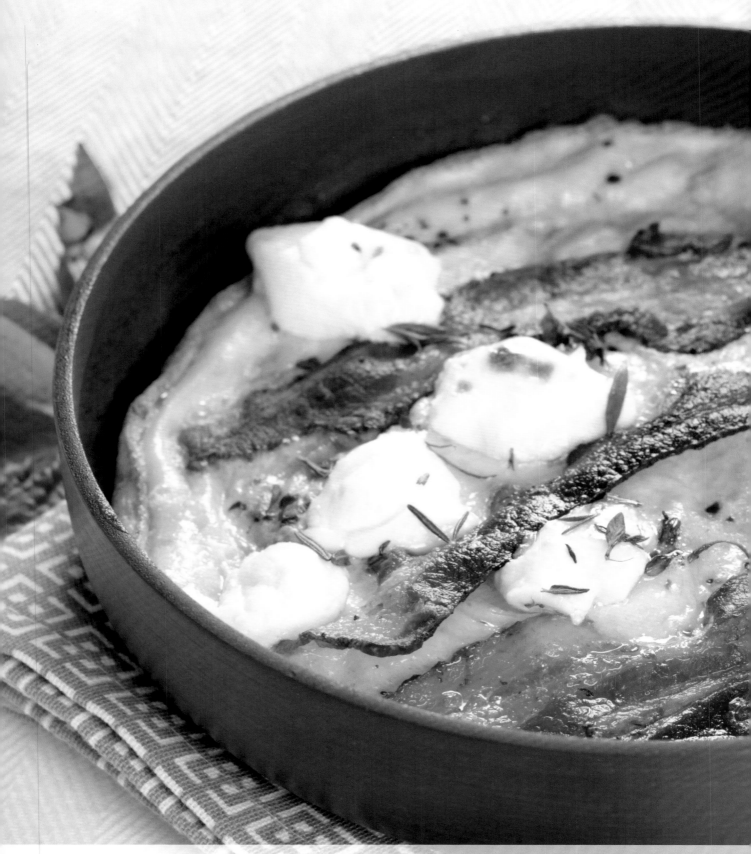

BACON AND CREAM CHEESE FRITTATA

Serves 4 | Ready in 35 minutes

4 pieces bacon
5g butter
6 eggs
80 mL water
5 mL oregano, ground
5 mL red pepper flakes
Dash of Tabasco sauce
100g cream cheese

PREHEAT oven to 175°C (350°F).

COOK bacon, and set aside. You may also chop cooked bacon up and add to egg mixture.

MELT butter in a cast iron skillet.

WHISK eggs, water, and spices together and pour into skillet.

PLACE into oven and bake for 20 minutes. Frittata will rise.

IN last 5 minutes, distribute bacon and cream cheese along the top of frittata. This will allow cheese and bacon to bake into frittata nicely.

REMOVE from oven and serve hot.

 The frittata will begin to fall once removed from the oven: try to serve while it's still fluffy!

NET CARBS 3.5G	PROTEIN 17.2G PER SERVING

GF

BREAKFAST FLATBREADS

Serves 8 | Ready in 30 minutes

95g almonds, ground
10g flaxseed, fresh ground
15g pecans, chopped
10g chia seeds, ground
15g hemp hearts
10g coconut flour
5 mL baking powder
2.5 mL salt
30 mL Alpha Balance™ Oil or camelina oil
2 eggs
100 mL quark (or sour cream)

PREHEAT oven to 175°C (350°F).

LINE a baking sheet with parchment paper.

COMBINE the first 8 dry ingredients. Add the oil, eggs and quark until well mixed.

USING a spatula, spread over the parchment-lined baking sheet, about 1cm thick. Another option for buns is to use a 2-inch ring mold and form rounds 1 cm thick.

BAKE for 20 minutes.

CUT into 8 equal pieces.

 These can be enjoyed many different ways! Try with a nut butter, homemade jam or with slices of avocado and tomato.

NET CARBS 2G	PROTEIN 6.9G PER SERVING

GF   VEG

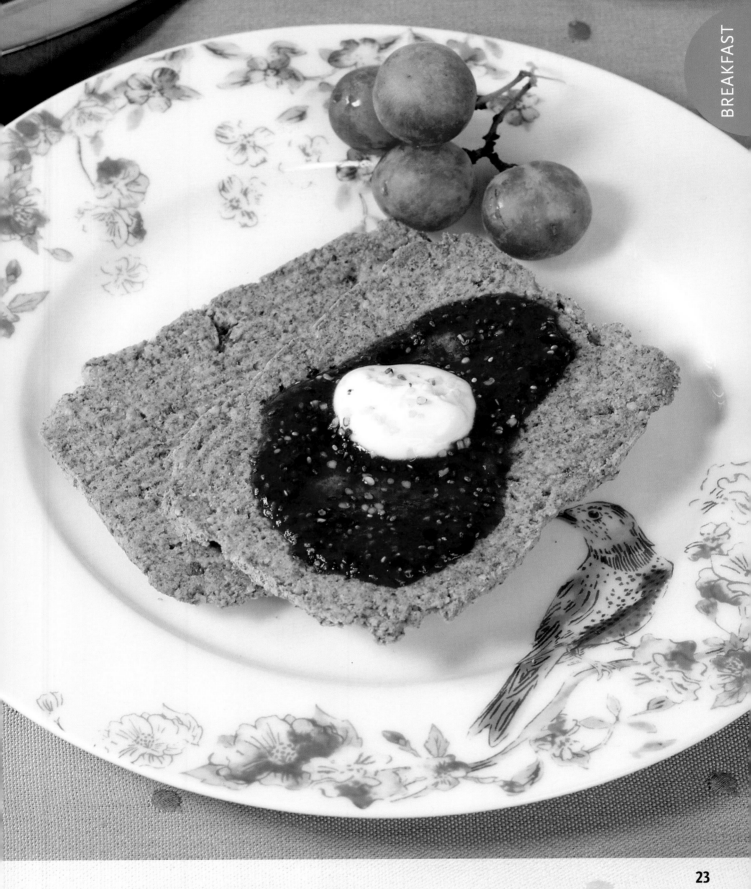

BREAKFAST FRUIT SALAD

Serves 4 | Ready in 15 minutes

200g avocado, peeled, pitted, diced

200g grapefruit, peeled, membrane removed, diced

200g papaya, peeled, seeded, diced

5 mL lime juice for salad

120g coconut cream, cold

2.5 mL lime juice for whip

½ lime, zested

60 mL Alpha Balance™ Oil

5g mint, chopped fine

This doesn't seem like much, but it's filling. If you're a morning coffee person, have this alongside one or two of the Apple Breakfast Muffins on page 18. —CG

GENTLY toss the papaya and avocado together in a medium bowl with the 5 mL of lime juice. Add grapefruit and toss again.

WHIP the coconut cream with the lime zest. When whipped, fold in the 2.5 mL lime juice.

DIVIDE the fruit salad into 4 bowls. Drizzle each bowl with 15 mL of oil. Sprinkle with chopped mint. Add a 30 mL dollop of lime coconut cream. Serve.

 If you want to make this the evening ahead, add a bit more lime juice to prevent the browning of the avocado, and cover in an airtight container. For a little bit of extra flavour, infuse the 60 mL of Alpha Balance™ Oil with some fresh mint or the contents of a peppermint teabag overnight.

NET CARBS 10G   PROTEIN 2.6G

 GF   VEGAN   DAIRY FREE   VEG

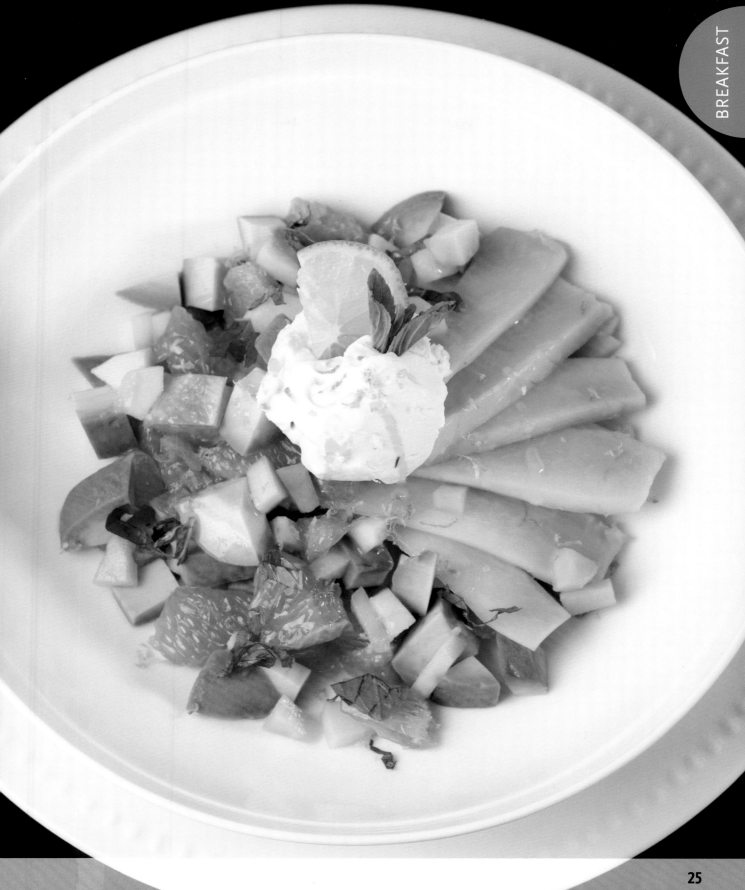

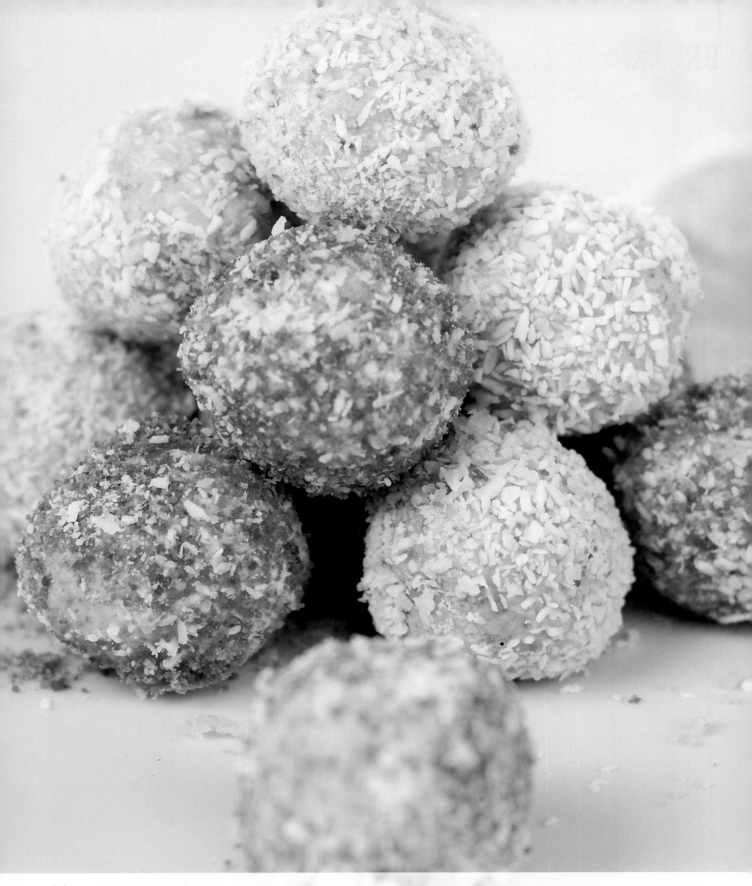

BREAKFAST TRUFFLES

Makes 20 truffles | Ready in 35 minutes

60g coconut flour
125 mL DME™ Coconut Oil, melted
120g cashews
30 mL lemon rind
30 mL vanilla
2.5 mL sea salt
12g coconut sugar (reserve half for coating)
Flaked coconut

The fresh lemon flavour will brighten even the dreariest of mornings. —AT

PLACE first 6 ingredients with half the sugar in a food processor and pulse until well combined.

REFRIGERATE mixture for 30 minutes to set.

ROLL a tablespoon of the truffle mixture into a ball and coat in flaked coconut and/or remaining coconut sugar.

STORE in the refrigerator in an air tight container.

 TIP Pre-make these and freeze for busy mornings or snack attacks.

NET CARBS 3.4G   PROTEIN 1.8G PER TRUFFLE

 GF   VEGAN   DAIRY FREE   VEG

CAULIFLOWER & MUSHROOM BISCUITS

Makes 12 biscuits | Ready in 1 hour

670g cauliflower florets
30 mL DME™ Coconut Oil
6g (2 cloves) garlic, minced
60g mushrooms, chopped fine
60g red bell pepper, chopped fine
2 eggs
20g coconut flour
30g hazelnuts, ground
5g chives, chopped
30 mL red pepper flakes (optional)
5 mL paprika

2.5 mL sea salt
2.5 mL pepper

PREHEAT oven to 205°C (400°F).

PULSE cauliflower in a food processor until it reaches a rice-like consistency.

SAUTÉ cauliflower with coconut oil, garlic and mushrooms. Cool.

ADD all remaining ingredients and stir until everything is well combined.

FORM thick, 3-inch round patties using ¼-cup scoops of batter, and place on a parchment-lined baking sheet.

BAKE for 35–40 minutes.

COOL 5 minutes before handling.

NET CARBS 2.5G	PROTEIN 3G PER BISCUIT

GF   VEG   DAIRY FREE

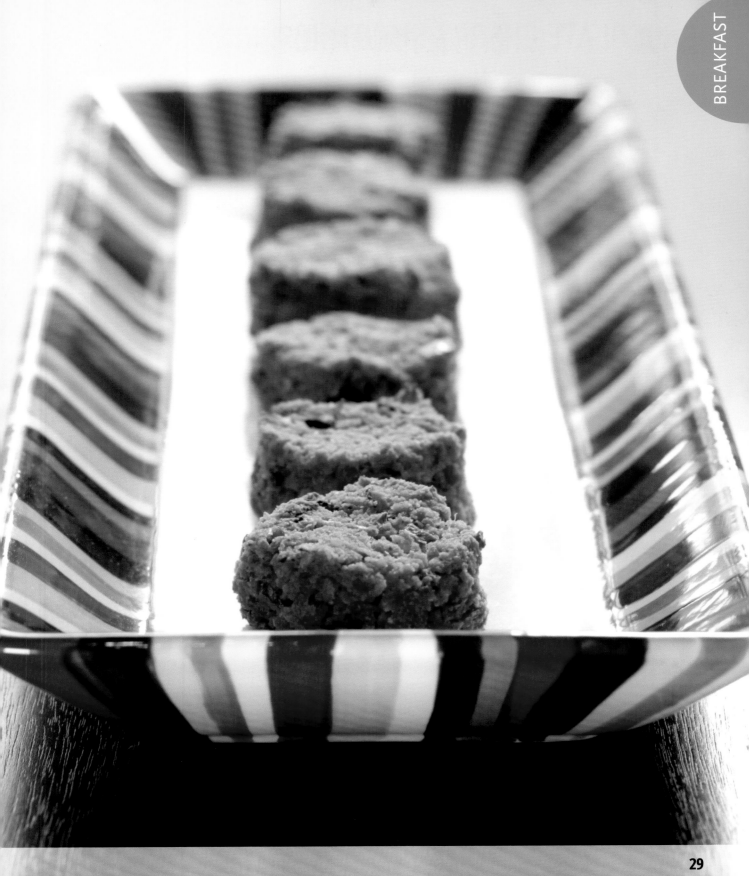

CHOCOLATE CHERRY SMOOTHIE

Serves 2 | Ready in 5 minutes

100g sour cherries, frozen
190 mL kefir (plain)
250 mL unsweetened almond milk
30g hemp hearts
30g flaxseed, fresh ground
30 mL Alpha Balance™ Oil
20g cacao or cocoa powder
5 mL vanilla
4 drops liquid stevia (optional)
1 pinch of sea salt

Fibre, anti-oxidants and healthy fats in five minutes flat. —AT

COMBINE everything in a high speed blender and serve.

NET CARBS 12.5G	PROTEIN 12.5G PER SERVING

GF   VEG

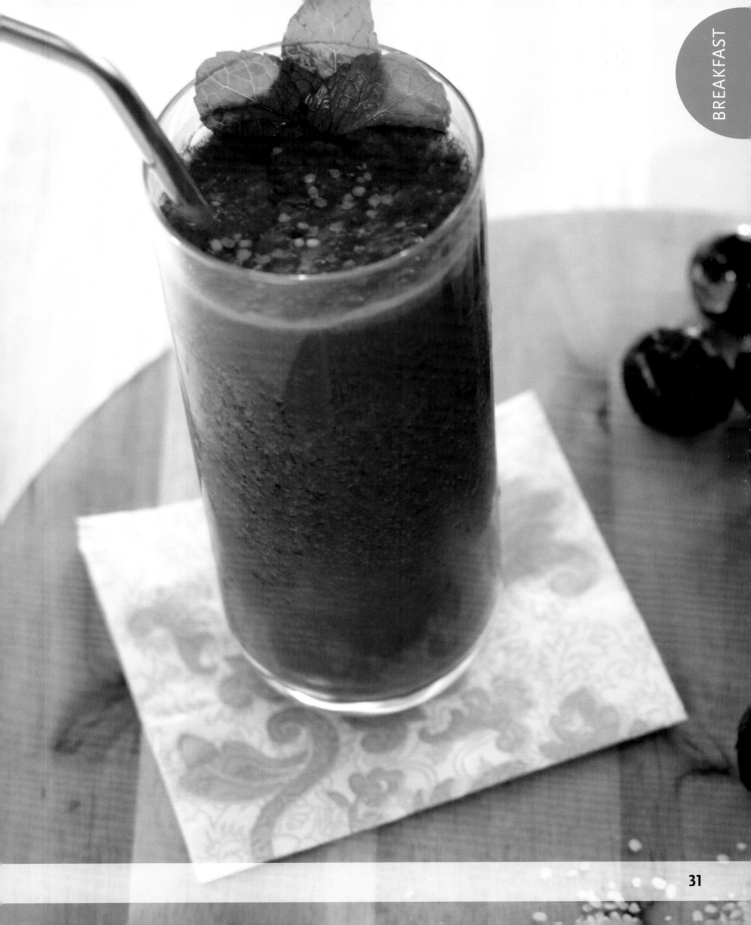

CRÊPES FLORENTINE

Serves 2 | Ready in 25 minutes

10g onion, chopped fine

4g garlic cloves,

100g spinach, chopped fine

60 mL heavy (whipping) cream

60 mL white wine or vermouth

30g grated Gruyère, Gouda or aged Cheddar

20g cranberries, fresh or frozen, chopped

15g flaxseed, fresh ground

15 mL Alpha Balance™ Oil

½ lemon, zested

5 mL lemon juice

Salt to taste

Pinch of white pepper

2 eggs, poached

2 Garbanzo Bean And Chestnut Crêpes
  (see page 39)

I love the addition of the cranberries, as they add brightness to the dish, and "take it over the top". The crêpe is a nice addition for presentation, but this could also be served with Breakfast Flatbreads (page 22), baked English muffin style. —CG

CHOP cranberries into ¼-inch pieces. Cook in a small pan over low heat with the wine to soften, about 10–15 minutes. All the liquid should be cooked off.

HEAT oil in pan over medium low. Add onions and sauté until soft. Add garlic and sauté until fragrant. Add spinach, sauté to wilt.

ADD cream and bring to simmer. Turn heat to low, stir in ground flaxseed. Add cheese slowly, stirring to combine.

STIR in the cooked cranberries. Add salt and white pepper to taste. Keep warm.

IN a separate pan, on low heat, warm crêpes.

WHILE crêpes are warming, poach eggs, then drain and blot. Place crêpes on warm plates.

DIVIDE mixture between crepes, reserving two tablespoons. Fold crêpe edges up to make pouch.

PLACE the poached egg on top of the crêpes.

GARNISH with balance of mixture and serve.

NET CARBS 8.5G	PROTEIN 14G PER SERVING *(FILLING ONLY)*
NET CARBS 11.9G	PROTEIN 16.1G PER SERVING *(INCLUDING CRÊPE)*

GF   VEG

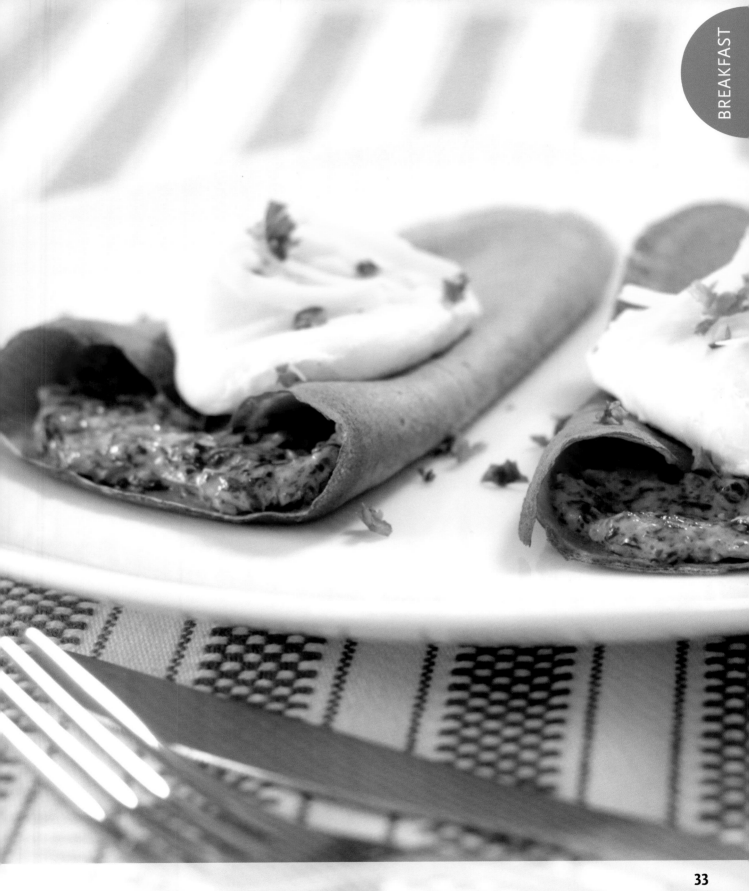

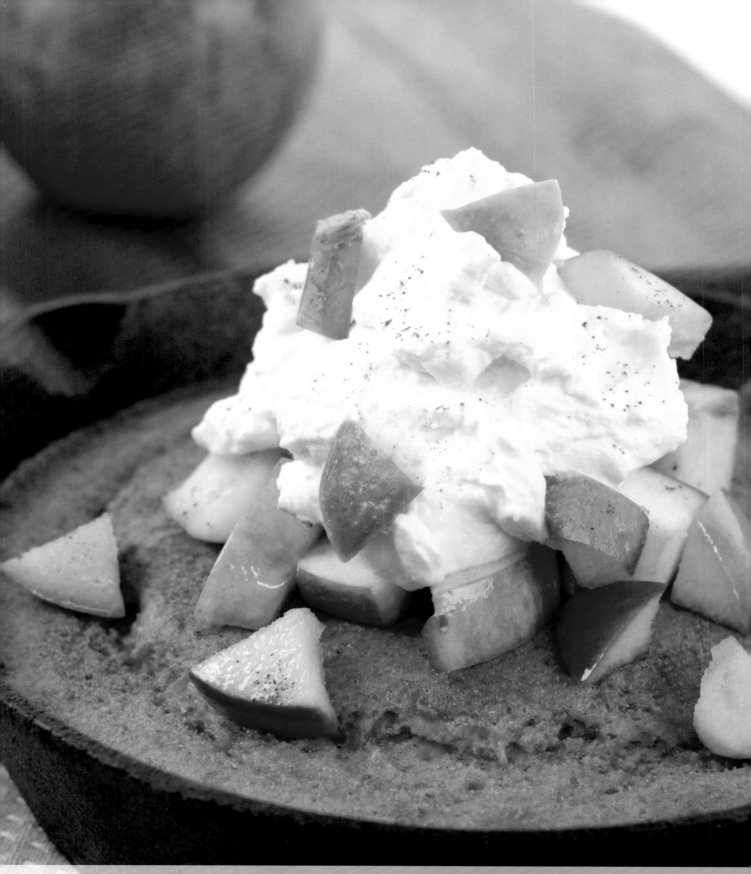

DUTCH BABY with Spiced Whipped Cream

Serves 4 | Ready in 30 minutes

DUTCH BABY

5 mL butter or DME™ Coconut Oil for pan
4 eggs
250 mL milk or milk alternative (almond works well)
10 mL vanilla extract
12g coconut sugar
30g coconut flour, sifted
5 mL baking powder
2.5 mL sea salt
5 mL cinnamon
200g fresh apple, cored, chopped into chunks

SPICED WHIPPED CREAM

125 mL heavy (whipping) cream
6g coconut sugar (optional)
5 mL vanilla
Pinch of cinnamon, clove and nutmeg

This delightful take on the apple pancake is perfect for 4 people and easily made dairy-free. – AT

DUTCH BABY

HEAT oven to 190°C (375°F).

BEAT eggs until fluffy in the bowl of a standing mixer.

ADD milk, vanilla and coconut sugar.

IN a separate bowl, sift remaining dry ingredients.

MIX dry with wet ingredients until just incorporated.

FOLD apple into batter.

GREASE cast iron pan or pie dish.

EVENLY pour batter into pan and cook until top is firm to touch and bottom is golden, about 20 minutes.

SERVE with spiced whipped cream!

SPICED WHIPPED CREAM

BEAT all ingredients on high until light and fluffy, and serve.

 Drizzle with maple syrup if you have little ones sharing your pancake!

NET CARBS 15.9G	PROTEIN 10G PER SERVING

 GF   VEG

EGGS BENEDICT

Serves 4 | Ready in 15 minutes

HOLLANDAISE SAUCE

70g butter
2 egg yolks
2.5 mL lemon zest
15 mL hot water
5 mL lemon juice
Pinch of paprika
Dash of cayenne
Salt to taste
5g fresh basil, chopped

15 mL vinegar
4 eggs
80g tomato, sliced
100g avocado, mashed
4 Breakfast Flatbreads (page 22)

HEAT water until bubbles form in a shallow pot. Melt butter in small stainless bowl over top (as a double boiler). Add the yolks as the butter melts and whisk with the whip attachment of an immersion blender. Add the lemon zest, and the hot water. As the sauce thickens, add the lemon juice. Keep blending constantly, about 10 minutes. When the sauce is thick, blend in the paprika, cayenne, and salt to taste.

IN another pan, heat water to near boiling. Add vinegar.

GENTLY crack eggs into the hot water. Poach eggs for 3 minutes.

TOAST flatbreads. Spread avocado, place tomato slice, then poached egg. Top with hollandaise sauce and garnish with fresh basil and serve.

 Making hollandaise sauce is an art, but it's worth learning. Temperature is the most important part of the process. If the sauce gets too hot, the proteins denature and the sauce breaks (it curdles and separates). If it doesn't get hot enough, it doesn't thicken. Lifting the bowl out of the water is a way of controlling the heat. If you see signs of curdling, remove the bowl from the heat immediately and throw in some ice chips. Keep blending. Even if the sauce breaks, it's still tasty; it just doesn't present as well.

NET CARBS 5G   PROTEIN 9.4G PER SERVING

GF   VEG

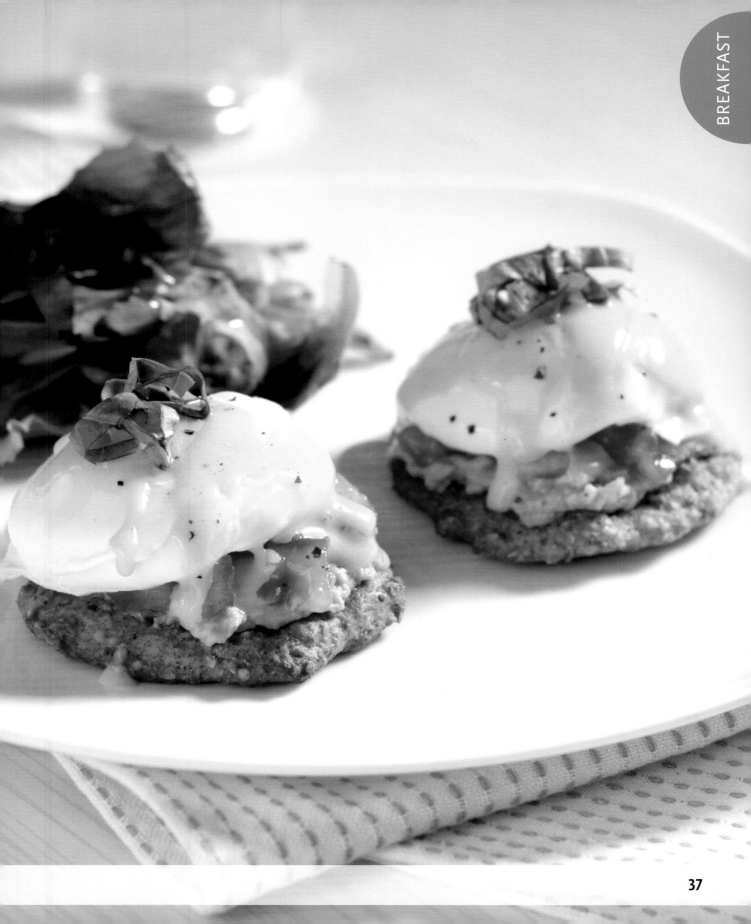

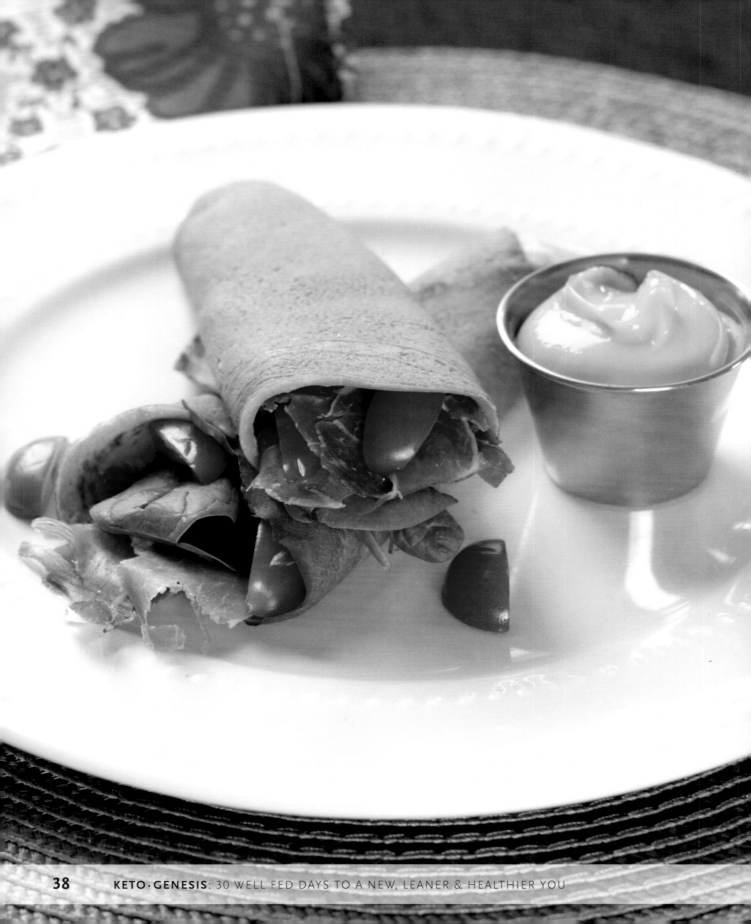

GARBANZO BEAN AND CHESTNUT CRÊPES

Serves 9 | Ready in 25 minutes

1 egg

125 mL milk

45 mL water

35g garbanzo bean flour

25g chestnut flour

Pinch of salt

15 mL butter, melted

COMBINE all ingredients in a blender or whisk by hand.

HEAT lightly greased skillet to medium high heat. Pour batter to thinly coat the bottom of the pan. Cook for 1 to 1 ½ minutes on the first side until golden. Flip and cook the second side for another 30 seconds.

MAKES 9 (8-inch) crêpes.

NET CARBS 3.4G	PROTEIN 2.1G PER CRÊPE

 GF   VEG

GREEK SALAD SCRAMBLE

Serves 2 | Ready in 20 minutes

4 eggs
75 mL water
5 mL crushed red pepper flakes
Pinch of salt and pepper
5 mL butter
50g grape tomatoes, halved
50g red onion, diced
50g red bell pepper, diced
100g spinach, chopped
5g fresh oregano
5g fresh thyme
50g sheep feta
10 kalamata olives, pitted, chopped
Sea salt and pepper to taste

This recipe gets a nice dose of vegetables into your day, and it is good for any meal of the day. — AT

WHISK eggs with water until uniform; season eggs with salt, pepper, and crushed red pepper.

HEAT a skillet on medium heat, add butter and melt.

ADD all vegetables and sauté for 3 minutes until soft.

ADD eggs, stir and cook until desired consistency is achieved.

FOLD in feta, olives and fresh herbs.

SEASON again with salt and pepper, and plate.

 If you have a Mediterranean store nearby you can stock up on lovely staples like olives, cheese, legumes and spices for future meals.

NET CARBS 8.3G	PROTEIN 19G PER SERVING

GF   VEG

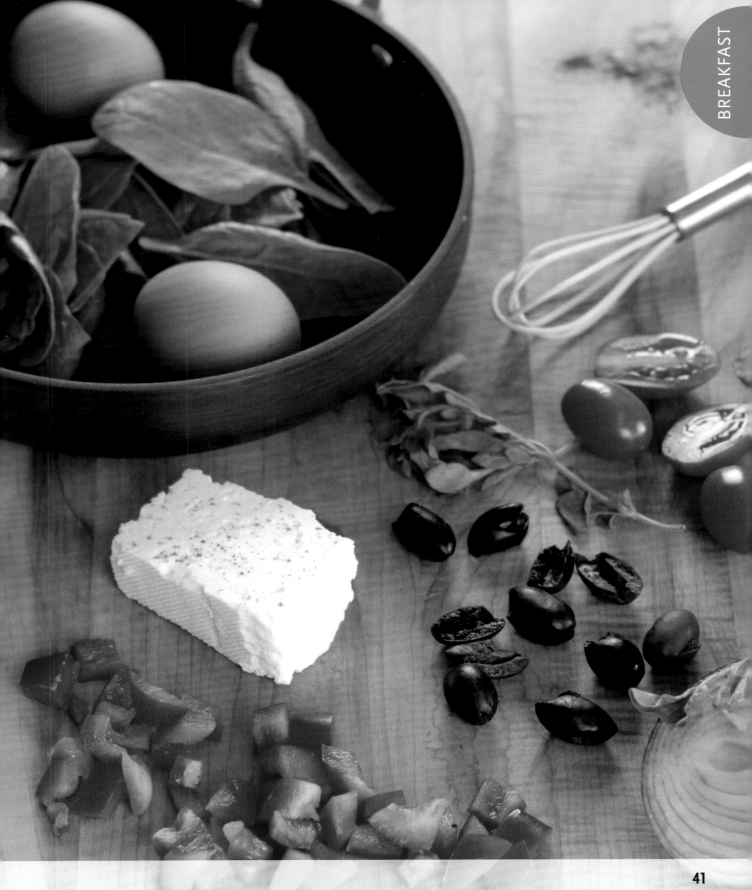

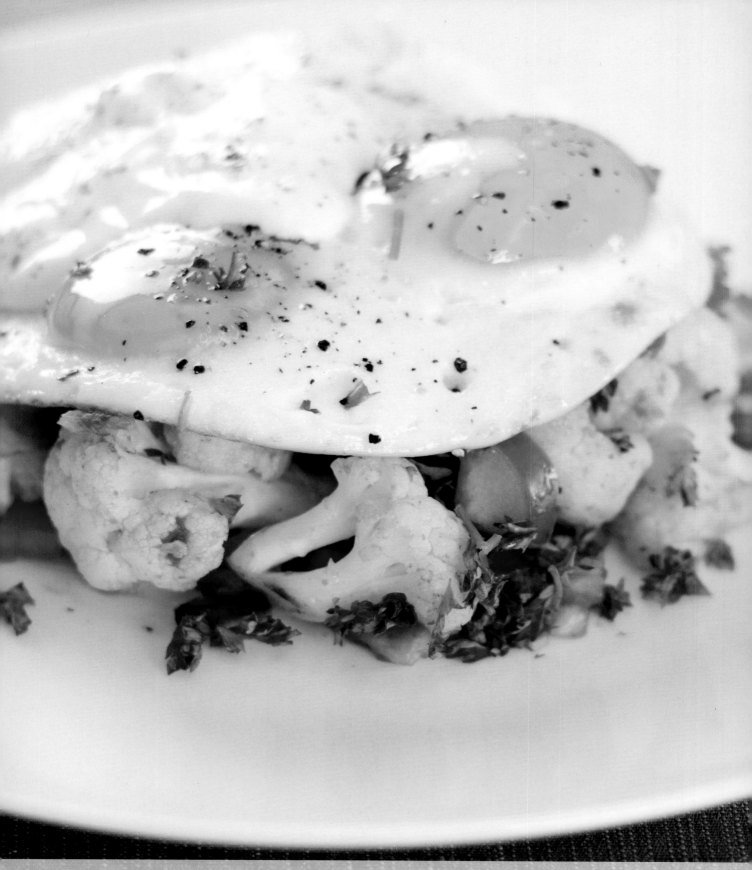

HARISSA CAULIFLOWER HASH with Fried Eggs

Serves 4 | Ready in 20 minutes

60g butter

100g onion, diced

10g (3 cloves) garlic, chopped

500g (1 head) cauliflower, chopped into bite-size pieces

100g red bell pepper, diced

20g flat leaf parsley, chopped

5 mL harissa chili paste (garlic chili paste, sriracha, or red Thai curry paste will also work)

8 eggs

125 mL full fat yogurt

Salt and pepper to taste

You won't miss the potatoes with this lively hash! —AT

MELT 45g butter over medium high heat, add onions, garlic, cauliflower, and sauté until golden.

ADD red pepper and stir in harissa. Let cook for 3 minutes more.

IN a cast iron or non stick pan, heat remaining butter and fry eggs until desired style is reached (a runny yolk is healthier, and provides a sauce for the hash).

SCOOP cauliflower hash into shallow bowls, top with yogurt, parsley and fried eggs.

SEASON with salt and pepper.

NET CARBS 10.4G	PROTEIN 19.3G PER SERVING

 GF   VEG

HAZELNUT CRÊPES

Serves 6 | Ready in 40 minutes

CRÊPES

120g whole wheat flour
120g hazelnut flour
2.5 mL baking powder
1.25 mL baking soda
1.25 mL salt
250 mL milk
90 mL water
5 mL maple syrup
2 eggs
5 mL honey
7.5 mL vanilla extract
125 mL butter, melted

FILLING

20g cucumber, diced small
20g strawberries, diced small
10g blueberries, chopped
20g raspberries, chopped

IN a large bowl, combine dry ingredients and blend well.

IN a medium bowl, whisk together the liquid ingredients until smooth. Add to the dry ingredients and stir to blend, making sure there are no lumps.

HEAT lightly greased skillet to medium high heat. Pour batter to thinly coat the bottom of the pan. Cook for 1 to 1½ minutes on one side until golden. Flip and cook the second side for another 30 seconds.

MAKES 18 (8-inch) crêpes.

 Crêpes can be prepared ahead and refrigerated, or frozen and reheated. If you plan to do this, layer a slip of parchment paper in between.

NET CARBS 18G   PROTEIN 8.8G PER SERVING (3 CRÊPES)

VEG

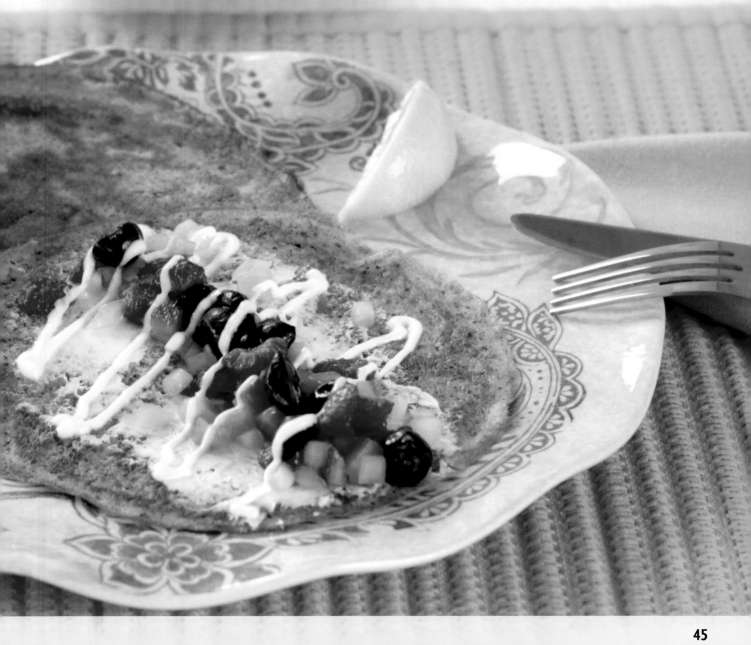

ITALIAN POACHED EGGS with Swiss Chard Nests

Serves 4 | Ready in 30 minutes

POACHING SAUCE

42g butter
9g (3 small) cloves garlic
425 mL (1 can) crushed tomatoes
25g fresh oregano leaves
25g fresh thyme leaves
1.25 mL crushed red pepper flakes
Salt and pepper to taste

8 eggs

SWISS CHARD NESTS

500g Swiss chard, rib removed and sliced
   into ribbons and steamed lightly for 2
   minutes.

50g fresh basil, shredded
90g fresh grated Parmesan

*A family and friend favourite, and brunch staple for many years.
— AT*

IN a medium pan, on medium heat, melt butter, add remaining sauce ingredients and purée with a hand mixer. Bring sauce to a gentle boil.

GENTLY crack eggs into sauce.

FORM Swiss chard into little nests, 1 per egg, on plates.

WHEN eggs reach desired doneness, gently scoop them out and place them in nests.

POUR a little bit of sauce over eggs, and sprinkle with cheese and basil. Serve immediately.

 You can make tomato sauce ahead of time and freeze until needed.

NET CARBS 10G	PROTEIN 23.5G PER SERVING

GF   VEG

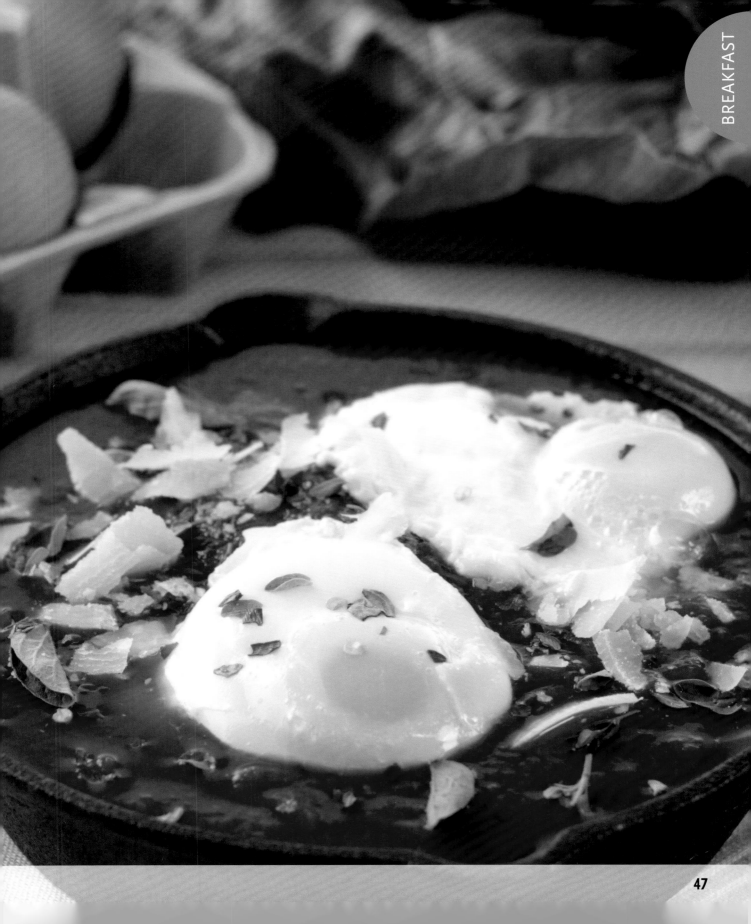

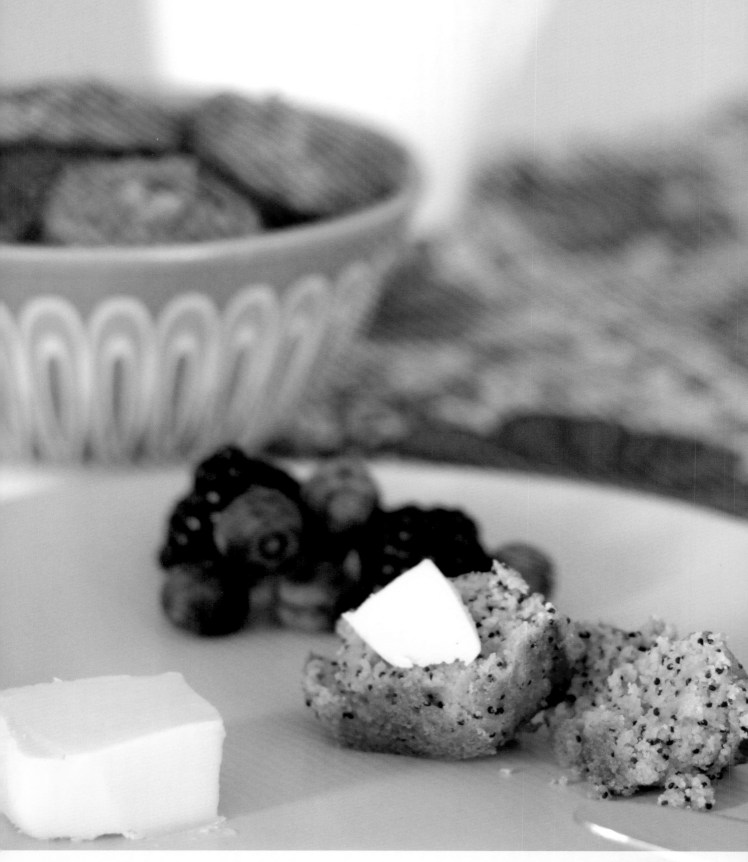

LEMON POPPYSEED MUFFINS

Makes 15 muffins | Ready in 35 minutes

15 mL lemon zest

16g poppy seeds

30g coconut flour

1.25 mL salt

1.25 mL baking soda

25 mL maple syrup

60 mL water

45 mL lemon juice

1 egg

22 mL DME™ Coconut Oil (melted and cooled)

These are great little grab-and-gos for breakfast. Combine two or three of them with an "Alpha Energizer" (page 18) for a quick, satisfying meal. —CG

PREHEAT oven to 175°C (350°F).

COMBINE lemon zest, poppy seeds, coconut flour, salt and baking soda in a medium bowl.

IN a separate bowl, combine maple syrup, water and lemon juice.

BEAT the egg until frothy in a third mixing bowl. Then add liquids, dry ingredients and coconut oil. Stir until moistened.

DROP into mini-muffin tins and bake for 18 minutes.

NET CARBS 2.5G   PROTEIN 1G PER MUFFIN

 GF   DAIRY FREE   VEG

NEAPOLITAN PARFAIT

Serves 4 | Ready in 15 minutes

120g cashews
100 mL boiling water
1.25 mL vanilla
5 mL DME™ Coconut Oil

120g avocado
20g medjool date
120g raspberries, fresh or frozen
5 mL lemon juice
20 mL water

120g dessert tofu
1.25 mL vanilla
15g cocoa powder

SOAK the cashews in boiling water. Set aside while preparing the rest of the parfait. Peel and seed the avocado. Seed and chop the medjool date finely. Add avocado, date, raspberries, lemon juice and water to food processor and purée. Use a spatula to scrape into bowl, and rinse out food processor.

COMBINE tofu, vanilla and cocoa powder in a food processor until smooth. Use spatula to scrape into bowl, and rinse out food processor for next step.

PURÉE cashews with soaking water in food processor. When smooth, add vanilla and coconut oil. Blend until smooth.

 TIP Layer cashew purée, chocolate purée, and top with raspberry purée. The chocolate is unsweetened, and provides a contrast to the cashews and raspberries.

NET CARBS 17G	PROTEIN 7.9G PER SERVING

 GF   VEGAN   DAIRY FREE VEG

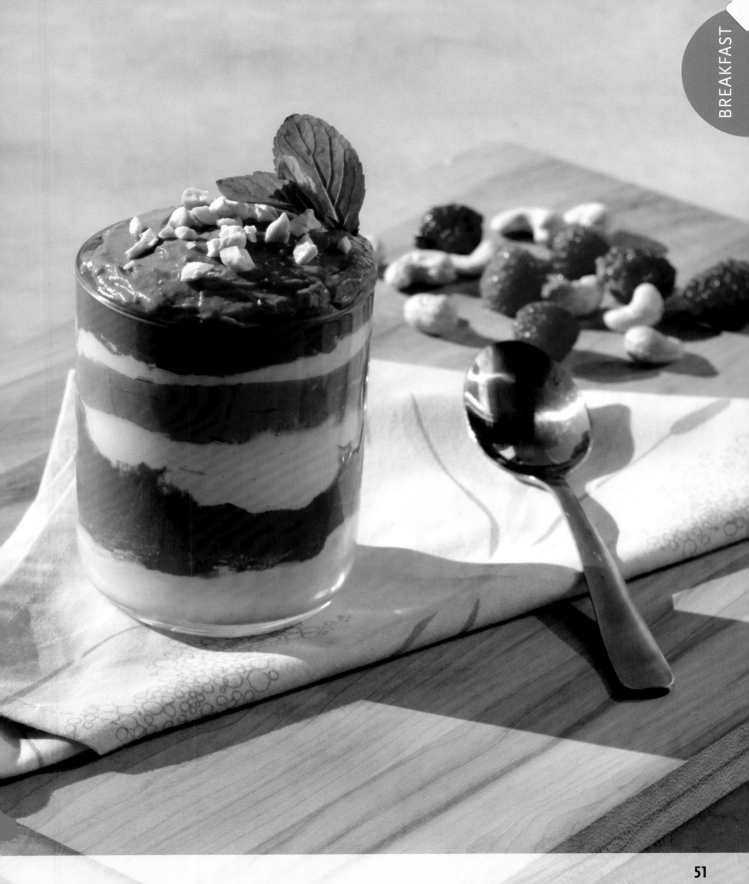

PERFECT COCONUT KETOGENIC OATMEAL

Serves 2 | Ready in 15 minutes

250 mL water
100g rolled oats
15 mL DME™ Coconut Oil
6g coconut sugar (optional)
2.5g cinnamon
Pinch of sea salt
15g unsweetened coconut flakes (optional)

Oatmeal just feels like a good start to a great day. – AT

BRING water to a boil and add oats, stirring continuously until water is just absorbed.

ADD coconut oil, and stir until incorporated into oats.

REMOVE from heat, place oats into a bowl, and top with coconut flakes.

 Serve with fresh fruit, like berries, and top with organic yogurt, almond milk or a touch of cream.

NET CARBS 32.2G	PROTEIN 7.8G PER SERVING

 VEGAN   DAIRY FREE   VEG

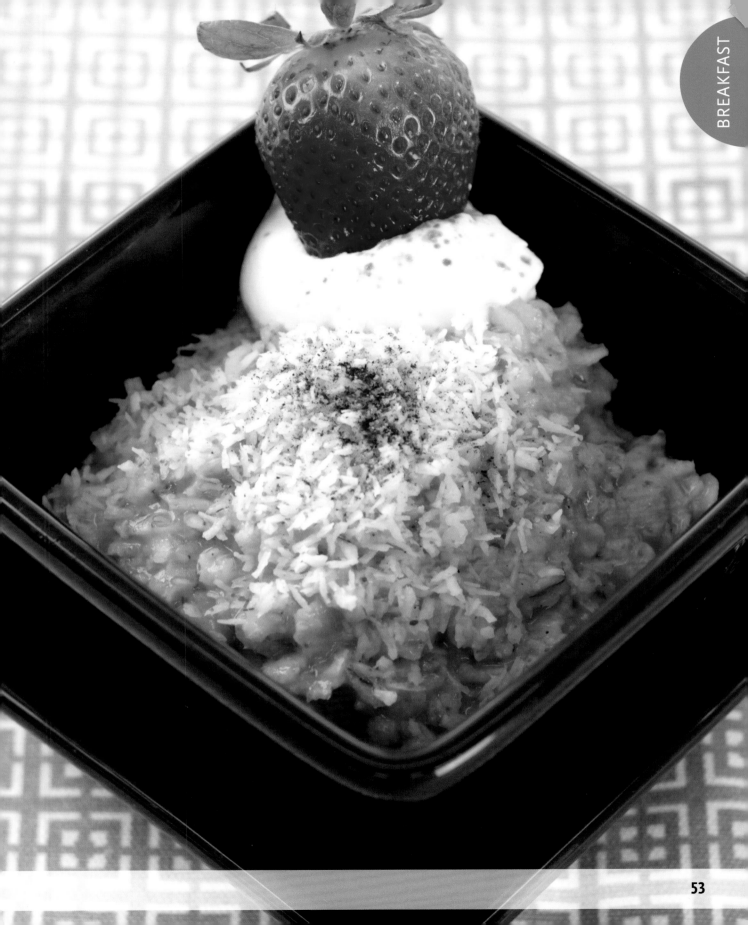

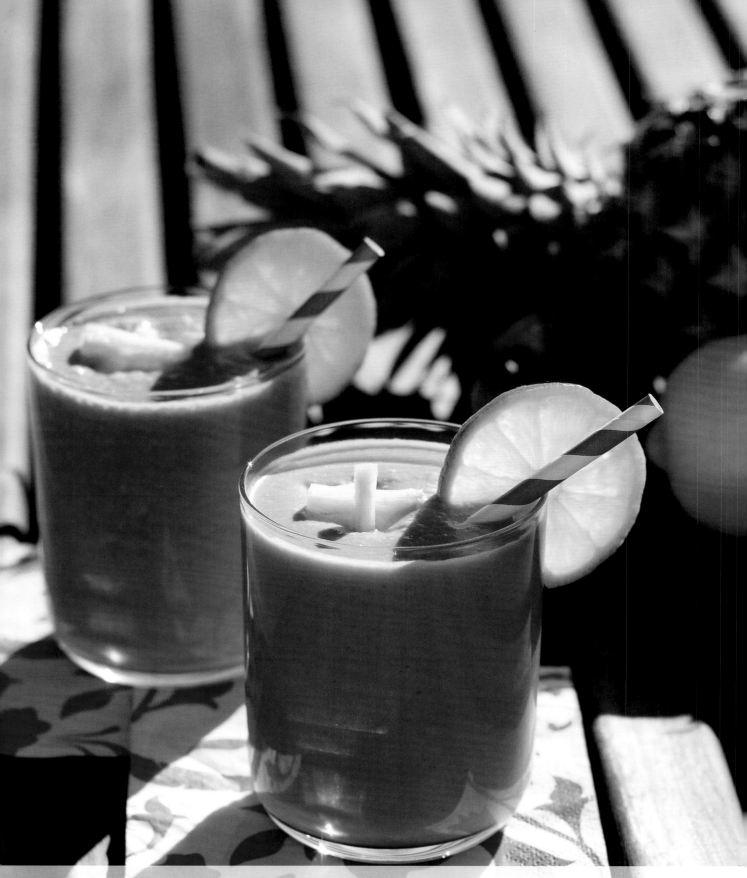

PIÑA COLADA SUPER GREEN SMOOTHIE

Serves 2 | Ready in 5 minutes

15 mL DME™ Coconut Oil

100g pineapple, fresh or frozen, diced

200g spinach, kale or swiss chard

250 mL coconut milk

60 mL lime juice

250 mL water

250 mL ice

This breakfast is refreshing and easy to make ahead, and you can sing that piña colada song as you make it – so there is really nothing to lose. – AT

BLEND until smooth. Enjoy.

 Some blenders may find greens to be a bit of a challenge. Try blending the spinach, kale or chard with your water first. Add remaining ingredients and blend until smooth.

NET CARBS 20.3G	PROTEIN 4.5G PER SERVING

 GF   VEGAN   DAIRY FREE   VEG

PUMPKIN AND BAKED APPLE "OATMEAL"

Serves 2 | Ready in 30 minutes

125g apple, chopped

15 mL butter, melted

425g (1 can) pumpkin purée (not pie filling)

250 mL half & half cream or almond milk

10g coconut flour

3g coconut sugar

2.5 mL each ground ginger, cinnamon,
   and clove

Pinch of sea salt

This pumpkin breakfast is similar to custard, and is loaded with fibre. Beautiful with berries and chopped pecans too. —AT

PREHEAT oven to 175°C (350°F).

TOSS apples in butter and bake on a parchment-lined cookie sheet until soft and golden, about 12 minutes.

REMOVE from oven and cool.

IN a sauce pan, add remaining ingredients, using a wire whisk to incorporate the flour into the cream and pumpkin evenly. Cook gently on low heat until thick.

ADD apples and serve.

NET CARBS 20.6G	PROTEIN 3.3G PER SERVING

 GF   VEG

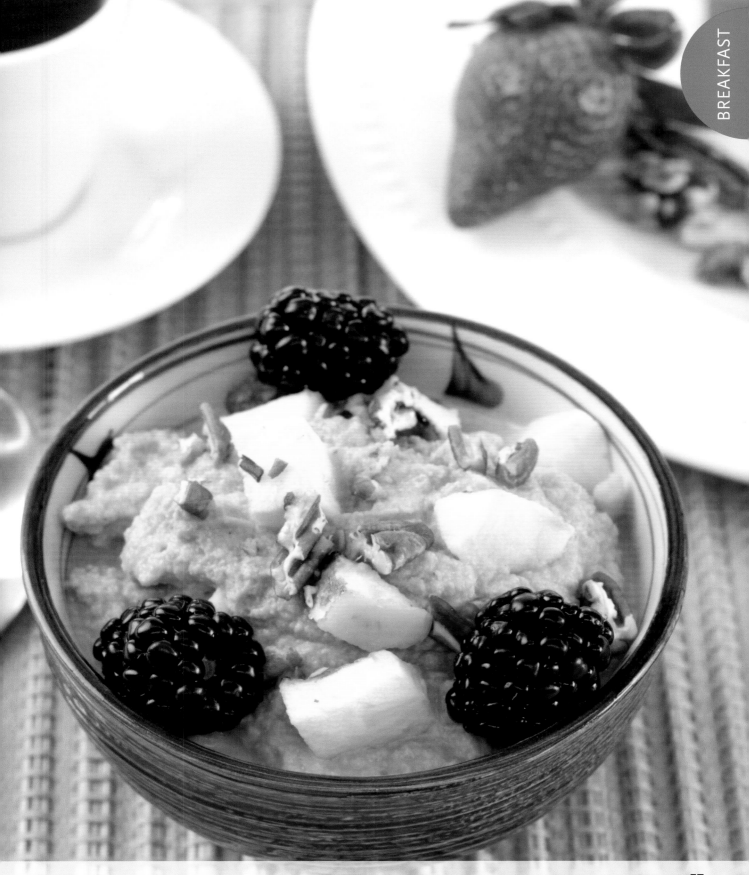

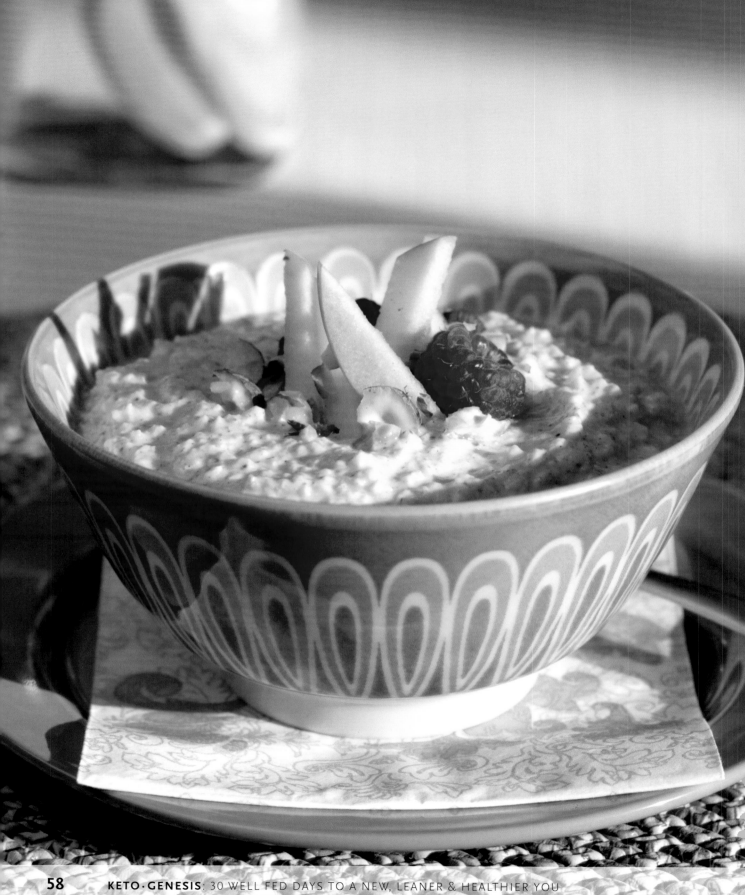

QUARK MUESLI

Serves 2 | Ready in 10 minutes

200g (2 small) Granny Smith apples
20 mL lemon juice
20g flaxseed, fresh ground
75g hazelnuts or pecans, ground
250g quark, clabbered cream or
    Greek (10% mf) yogurt
Pinch of cinnamon
Pinch of salt
30 mL Alpha Balance™ Oil
30 mL DME™ Coconut Oil, melted or
    camelina oil

Quark muesli was Dr. Johanna Budwig's standby for her cancer therapy. There's something about the combination of Omega 3 fatty acids and the sulphur rich proteins in the fermented milk products that produces magic in the human body. This is an updated variation on the recipe served at our breakfast table growing up, as well as every Alive Health Retreat my father, Siegfried, ever hosted. —CG

COMBINE apples and lemon juice in food processor and blend until fine.

ADD all other ingredients and combine until smooth.

 Quark is an unprocessed cottage cheese. It's sometimes hard to come by. Clabbered cream is making sour cream the old fashioned way, by letting milk sour. If you want to do it with today's pasteurized milk, you need to add something with culture, like yogurt, or cultured sour cream. Add a tablespoon or two per 250 mL. Let it stand in a slightly warmer than room temperature place for a day or two, and let the beneficial bacteria do their job. If you start with heavy cream, you end up with a nice, fatty, satisfying clabbered cream. Feel free to experiment with the different cultures as they'll give you different end flavours.

NET CARBS 18.5G   PROTEIN 20.8G PER SERVING

GF   VEG

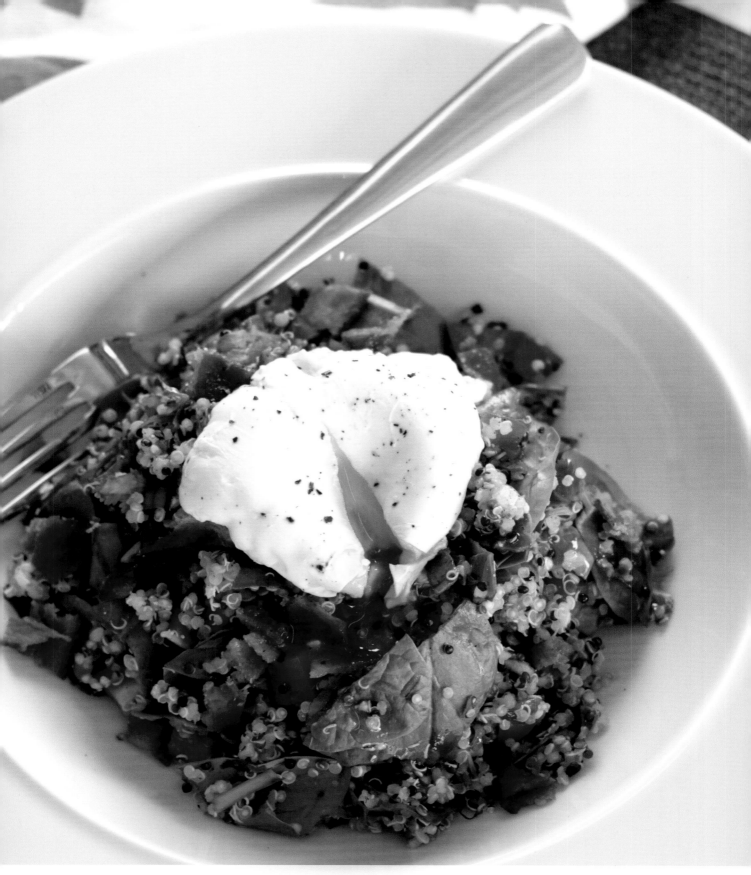

KETO·GENESIS: 30 WELL FED DAYS TO A NEW, LEANER & HEALTHIER YOU

QUINOA BREAKFAST SALAD

Serves 4 | Ready in 25 minutes

160g quinoa, cooked according to package
    directions

125g baby spinach, washed and dried, then
    roughly chopped

8 strips of bacon, cooked and crumbled

150g ripe avocado, chopped

100g red bell pepper, diced

100g chopped green onion

10g fresh cilantro

60 mL olive oil

45 mL lemon juice

4 eggs

You can make the base of the salad in advance, and warm up portions as needed and then top with a poached egg. Or, hard boil an egg, peel and add to salad before serving. – AT

IN a large bowl, combine all ingredients except the eggs and let marinate for a minimum of 20 minutes or let sit overnight.

SEPARATE into four servings.

TOP with a soft poached egg or hard-boiled egg.

NET CARBS 14.5G   PROTEIN 16.6G PER SERVING

GF   DAIRY FREE

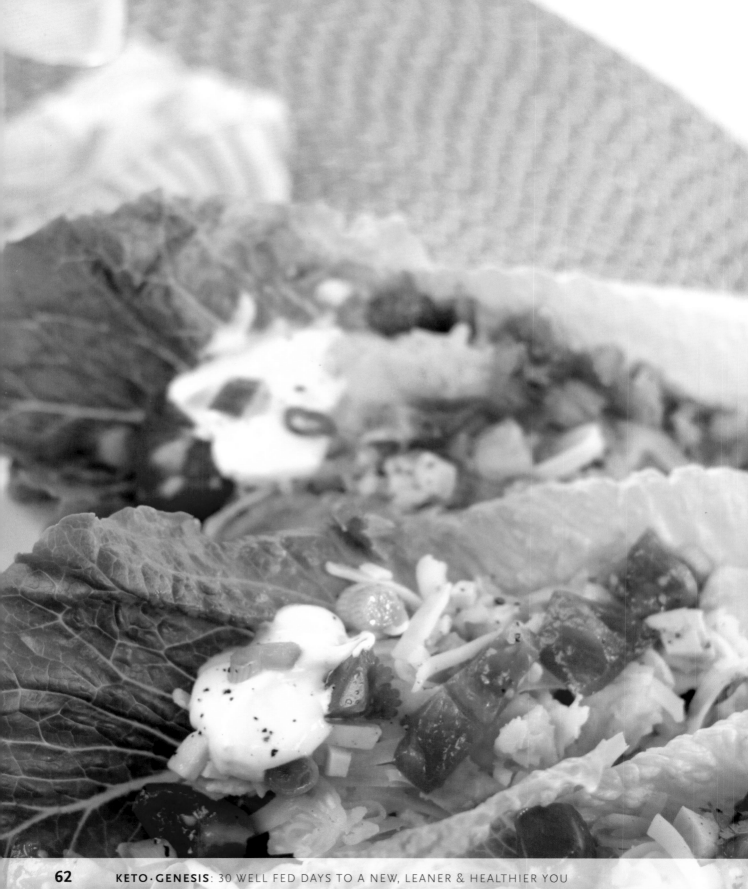

ROMAINE BREAKFAST BURRITOS with Quick Homemade Salsa

Serves 4 | Ready in 20 minutes

30g butter

6 eggs

60 mL water

20g cilantro, washed and rough chopped

100g medium Cheddar, grated

700g Romaine lettuce, large leaves, washed and patted dry

400g (2 large) avocados, diced

45 mL Greek (10% mf) yogurt

Salt and pepper to taste

Serve with Quick Homemade Salsa (recipe follows)

A quick breakfast, and children love it too! — AT

TURN burner on low heat and melt butter in a medium sized sauce pan.

WHEN butter is just melted, add eggs and water, and scramble mixture.

COOK eggs over low heat until whites are just firm. Add cilantro, salt and pepper and remove from heat.

PLACE washed romaine on plates and fill with eggs. Top with grated cheese, avocado, salsa and a dollop of Greek yogurt.

 Cooking eggs over high heat damages the omega 3 fats in the yolk. Eggs are most nutritious when soft boiled, poached, or soft scrambled.

NET CARBS 7G	PROTEIN 22.2G PER SERVING

GF   VEG

QUICK HOMEMADE SALSA

100g tomatoes, rough chopped (grape tomatoes work nicely)

15 mL lime juice

1.25 mL hot sauce

25g green onions, chopped

2g chopped cilantro

Salt and pepper to taste

MIX all ingredients together and let sit for a few minutes before serving.

NET CARBS 1.3G	PROTEIN .4G PER SERVING

GF   VEG

SIEGFRIED'S FRITTATA

Serves 4 | Ready in 45 minutes

4 eggs

60 mL heavy (whipping) cream

50g Gruyère, grated

50g old Cheddar, grated

3g oregano

1g fresh thyme

4g fresh basil

1g fresh tarragon

5g fresh chives

2.5 mL salt

Pepper to taste

15g butter

25g onion

7g (2 cloves) garlic, minced

15 mL Bragg's liquid soy seasoning

This was my father's favourite contribution to brunch. The frittata is always so nice and fluffy coming out of the oven. It does fall though, once it hits the cold air. Fortunately, that doesn't affect the flavour. If you have more people to feed, double the recipe and use a bigger pan. – CG

PREHEAT oven to 175°C (350°F).

BEAT eggs, add cream, cheese, herbs, Bragg's, salt and pepper. Stir well to combine.

IN a heavy 25cm pan (cast iron or stainless) over medium low heat, melt butter and sauté onions until soft. Add minced garlic and continue sautéing until fragrant.

ADD egg mixture to pan and cook to form slight crust on edges, about 3 minutes.

PUT pan in oven and bake until middle rises and is golden, about 25–30 minutes.

CUT and serve.

 TIP Frittatas can be made ahead and served cold or reheated the next day (do you think you're getting anything fresher at Starbucks?) for a quick grab-and-go breakfast. Still sooo tasty...

NET CARBS 2.7G	PROTEIN 14G PER SERVING

GF   VEG

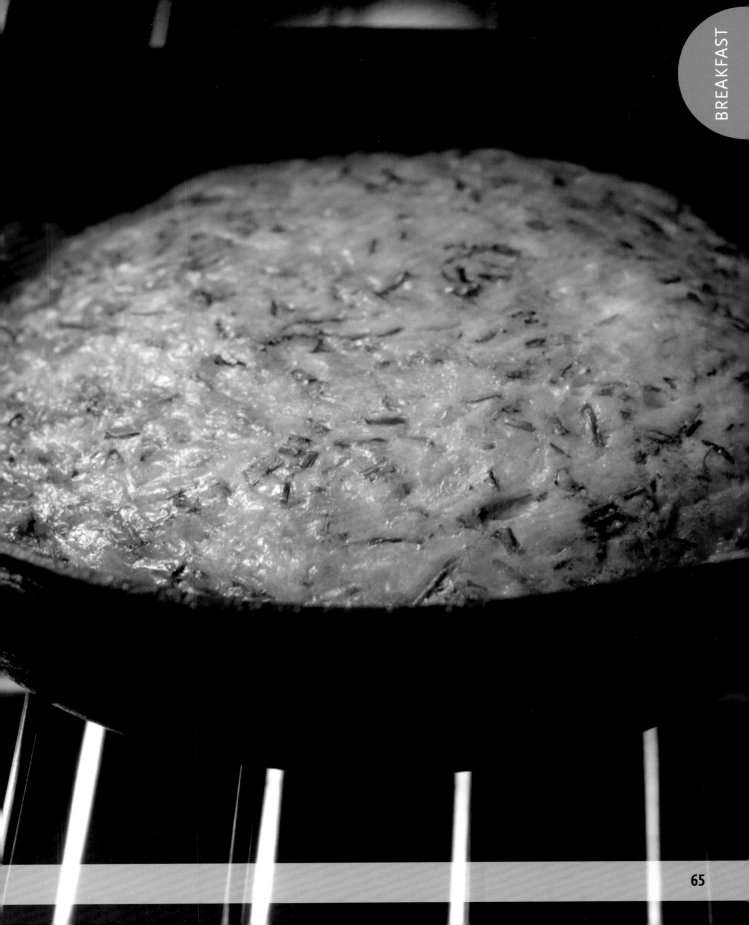

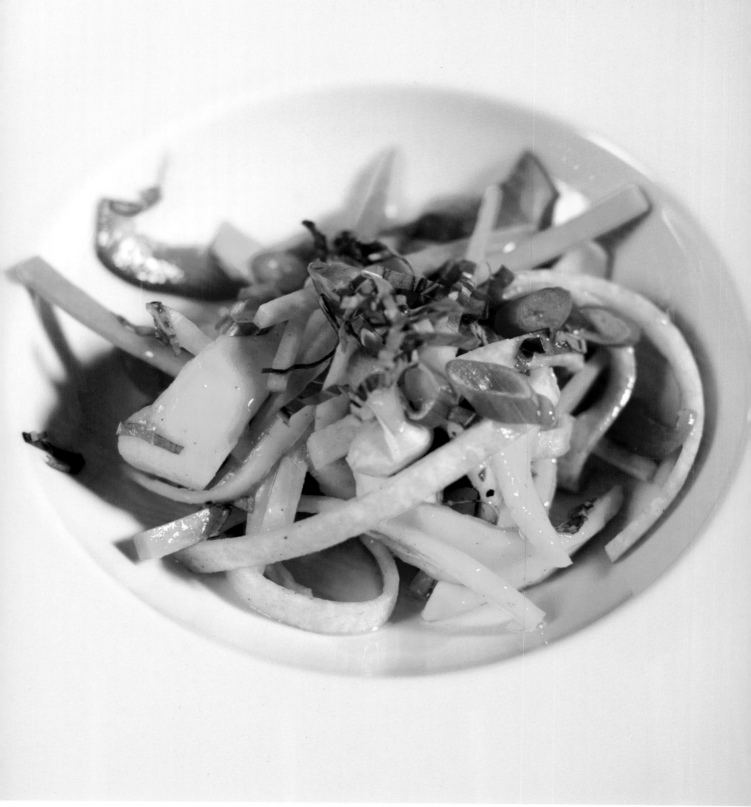

THAI GREEN MANGO SALAD

Serves 6 | Ready in 20 minutes

Pinch of coriander

Pinch of paprika

15g coconut sugar

30 mL lime juice

30 mL Alpha Balance™ Oil or camelina oil

30 mL Bragg's liquid soy seasoning

1 Thai chili, minced. Omit seeds and
   membrane to reduce heat

400g mango, julienned

200g jicama, julienned

200g red bell pepper, julienned

100g carrot, julienned

40g peanuts or cashews, chopped

30g green onions, fine sliced

20g fresh basil

COMBINE spices, sugar, lime juice, oil and Bragg's. Blend with a fork. Add Thai chili. Let sit to meld the flavours.

COMBINE sauce with julienned vegetables.

TOP with green onions, nuts, and basil just before serving. May be served immediately, or chilled overnight for breakfast.

 Green mangos are not always easy to find. This dish can be made with ripe mangos, but they don't julienne as easily. Just pick the firmest mango you can find, and do your best. The flavour is delicious, regardless.

NET CARBS 23G	PROTEIN 4.6G PER SERVING

 GF   VEGAN   DAIRY FREE   VEG

SWEET ACORN SQUASH PORRIDGE with Maple Bacon & Pecans

Serves 6 | Ready in 45 minutes

450g (1 large) acorn squash, halved,
    pulp and seeds removed
6 strips bacon
30 mL dark maple syrup
1.5 mL ground pepper
60g butter or DME™ Coconut Oil
2.5 mL cinnamon
2.5 mL ground ginger
2.5 mL ground cloves
125 mL cream or full fat coconut milk
14g coconut flour
50g raw pecans, chopped

This surprising breakfast hits all the right spots. – AT

PREHEAT oven to 205°C (400°F) and line 2 cookie sheets with parchment paper or a silicone mat.

PLACE acorn squash on first cookie sheet, cut side down, and cook until soft (30–40 minutes).

REMOVE from oven and let cool. Once cool, remove squash from skin.

USING second cookie sheet, toss bacon in maple syrup and sprinkle with ground pepper. Cook on each side for 10 minutes. Remove and cool on a wire rack.

MELT butter in a sauce pan over low heat. Add spices and warm for 2 minutes.

ADD squash, flour and cream, and purée with an immersion blender or whisk until blended.

TOP with candied bacon and pecans.

 Prepare the squash and bacon ahead of time, and refrigerate to make this a quick breakfast meal.

NET CARBS 13.7G   PROTEIN 5G PER SERVING

GF

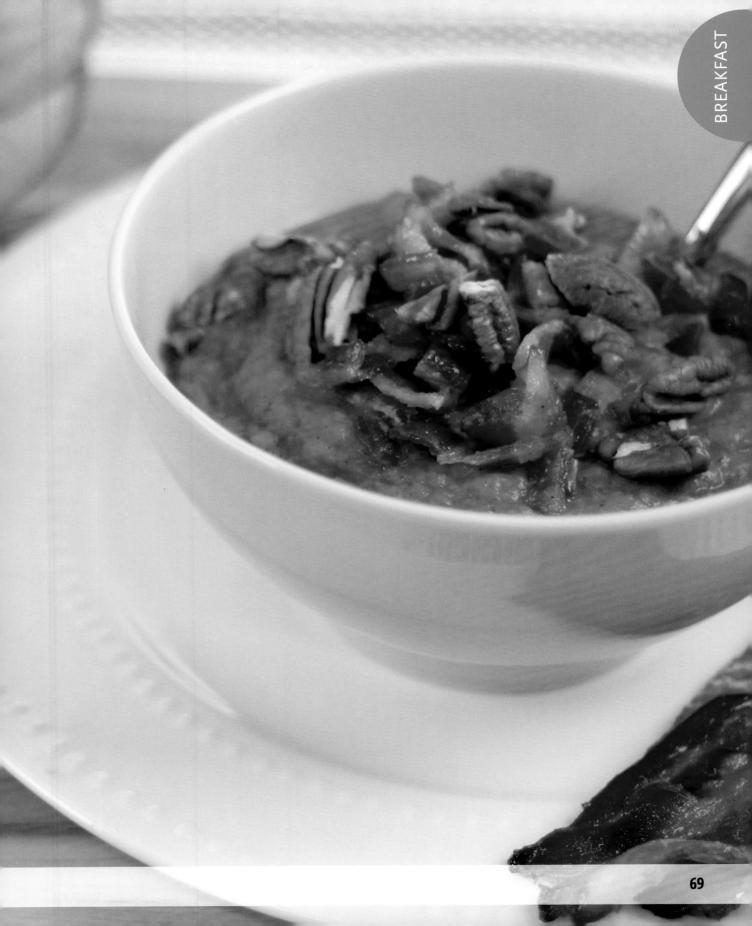

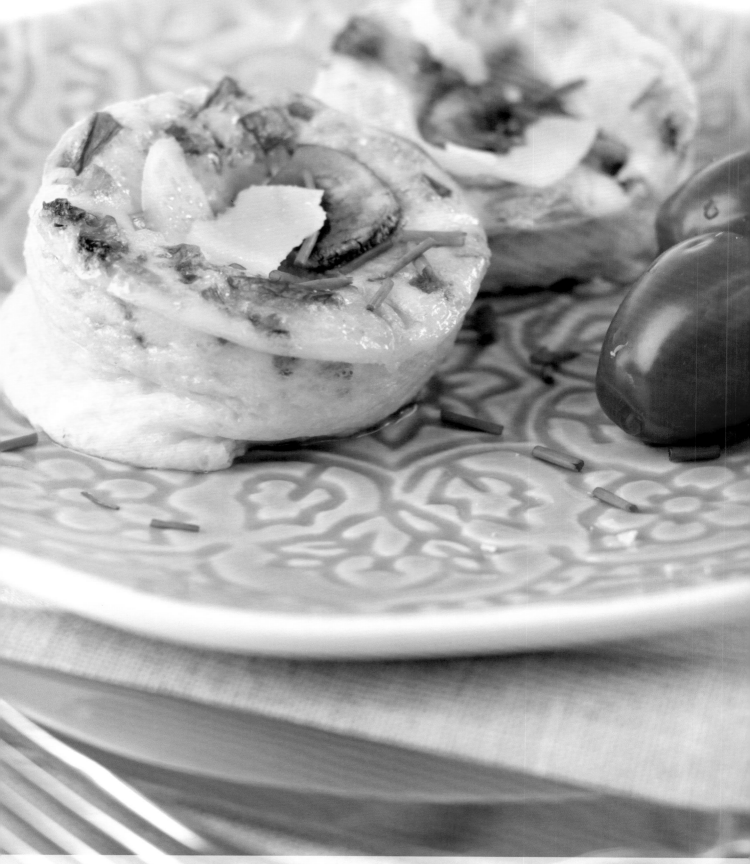

THREE CHEESE BREAKFAST BAKE

Serves 4 | Ready in 30 minutes

6 eggs

45 mL milk

2.5 mL smoked paprika

Fresh ground pepper and salt, to taste

50g Gruyère cheese

50g Parmesan cheese

50g Cheddar cheese

75g mushrooms, sliced or chopped

25g green onions, chopped

PLACE eggs, milk and spices into a bowl, and whisk.

FOLD in mushrooms, green onions, Cheddar and Gruyère.

POUR into a greased casserole dish or muffin tin and top with Parmesan cheese.

BAKE at 175°C (350°F) for 30 minutes for a casserole dish, and 15 minutes for muffin tins.

 Extras refrigerate wonderfully for perfect meals on the go!

NET CARBS 2.8G	PROTEIN 21.7G PER SERVING

GF VEG

VANILLA CHIA BREAKFAST PUDDING

Serves 4 | Ready in 1–4 hours

250 mL full fat yogurt

250 mL whole milk

90g black or white chia seeds

15g freshly grated lemon rind

12g coconut sugar

5 mL vanilla

150g strawberries, sliced

Perfect for breakfast on the go. Make a batch Sunday night for a yummy and healthy start to your week. —AT

MIX yogurt, milk, chia, sugar, lemon rind and vanilla in a blender, or whisk with a wire whisk. Refrigerate, stirring occasionally, for at least 1 hour, although 4 hours is perfect.

WHEN pudding is set, serve with fresh berries.

 Pudding can be made vegan by using 150g of soaked and rinsed cashews, and non-dairy milk of your choice.

NET CARBS 4G	PROTEIN 20.8G PER SERVING

GF   VEG

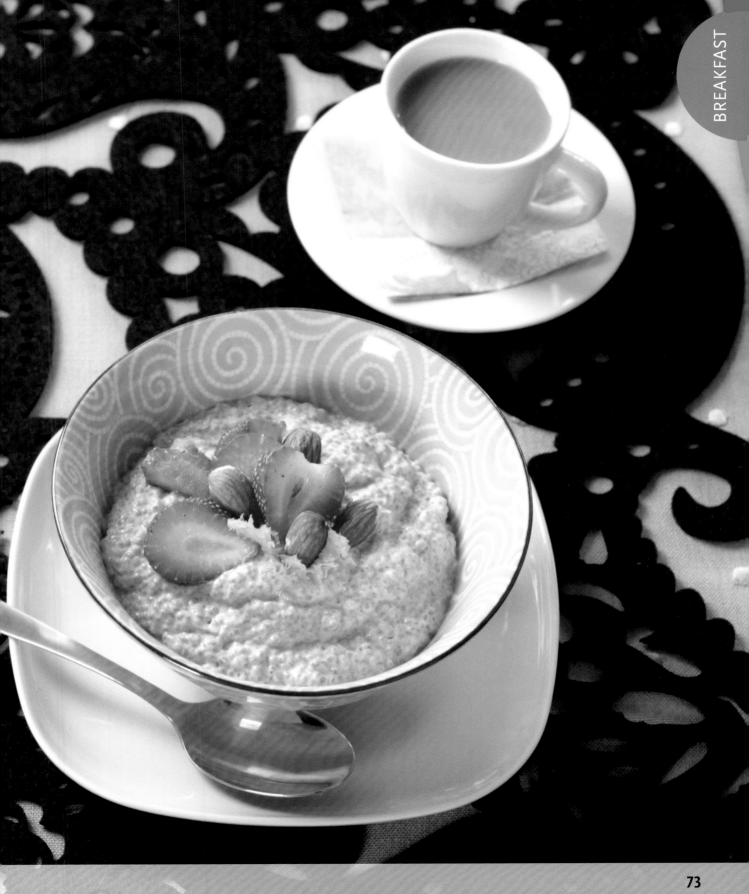

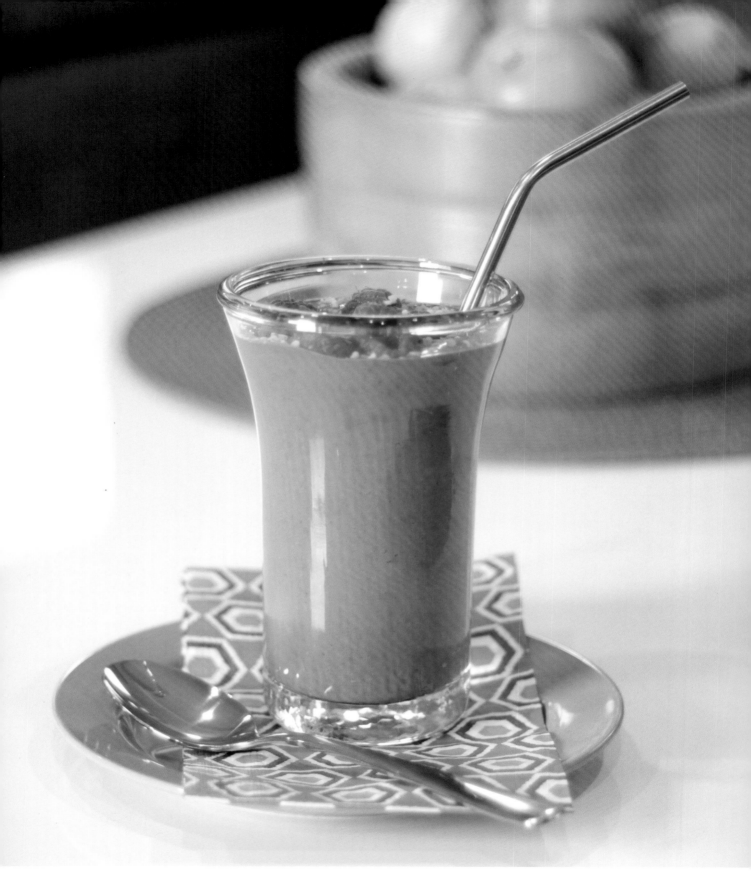

VEGAN CHOCOLATE AVOCADO SMOOTHIE

Serves 2 | Ready in 5 minutes

200g frozen banana

200g avocado

30g spinach

15 mL DME™ Coconut Oil

5g cacao powder or cocoa powder

2.5 mL vanilla extract

500 mL unsweetened almond milk

250 mL ice, optional

Cacao powder is raw cocoa – you can find it in most health food shops or organic grocers. It is loaded with nutrients and flavour! –AT

IN a high powered blender, blend all ingredients until smooth and creamy.

 If you are working with a standard kitchen blender, blend the spinach with the almond milk first, then add remaining ingredients.

NET CARBS 24G	PROTEIN 5G PER SERVING

 GF   VEGAN   DAIRY FREE   VEG

VEGAN GRANOLA

Serves 4 | Ready in 5 minutes

100g walnuts, chopped
40g flaxseed, fresh ground
20g chia seeds, fresh ground
10 mL vanilla bean powder
30g goji berries
Pinch of sea salt
50g fresh blueberries
25g fresh raspberries
250 mL unsweetened almond milk

This recipe is full of fibre and omega 3s. — AT

TOSS all ingredients and serve with almond milk.

 Pre-mix dry ingredients for granola and store in the fridge for an easy grab-and-go breakfast.

NET CARBS 9.8G	PROTEIN 8.5G PER SERVING

 GF   VEGAN   DAIRY FREE   VEG

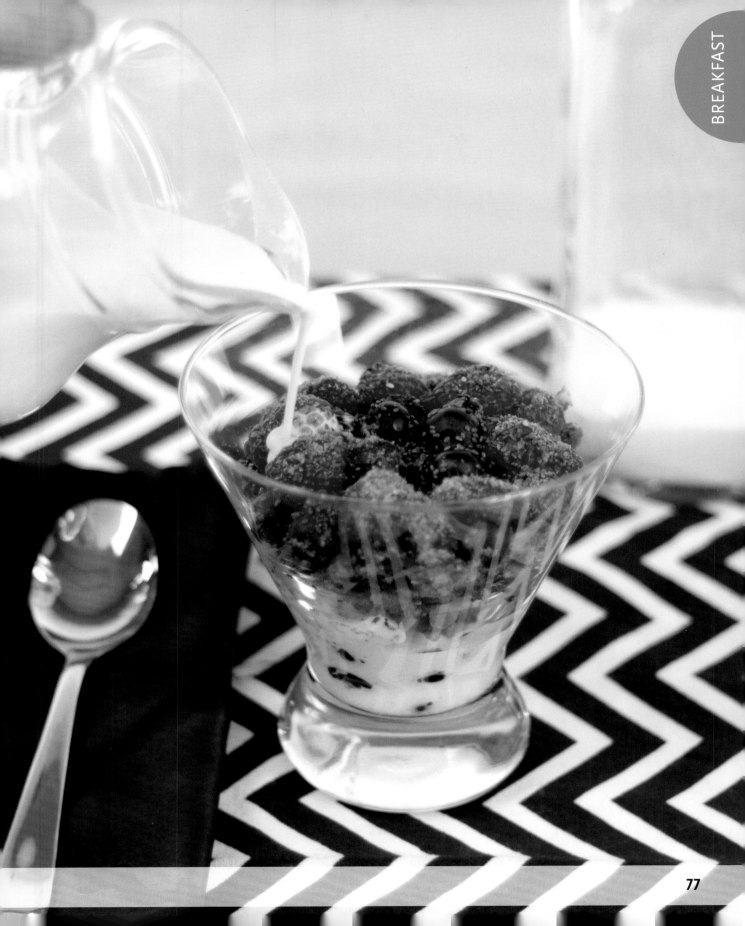

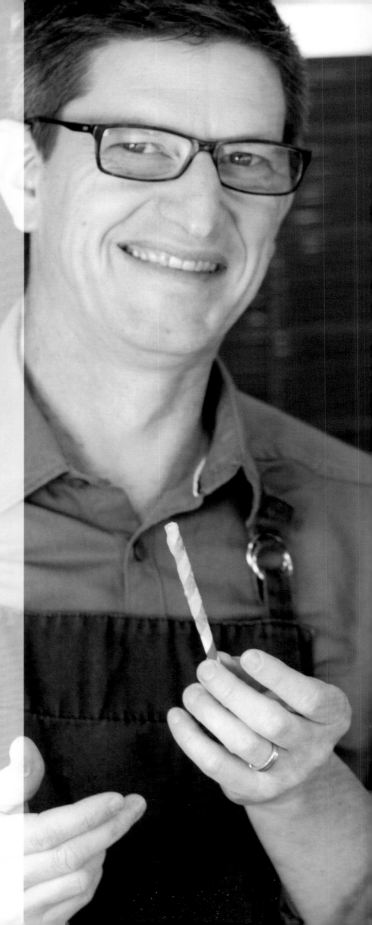

LUNCH

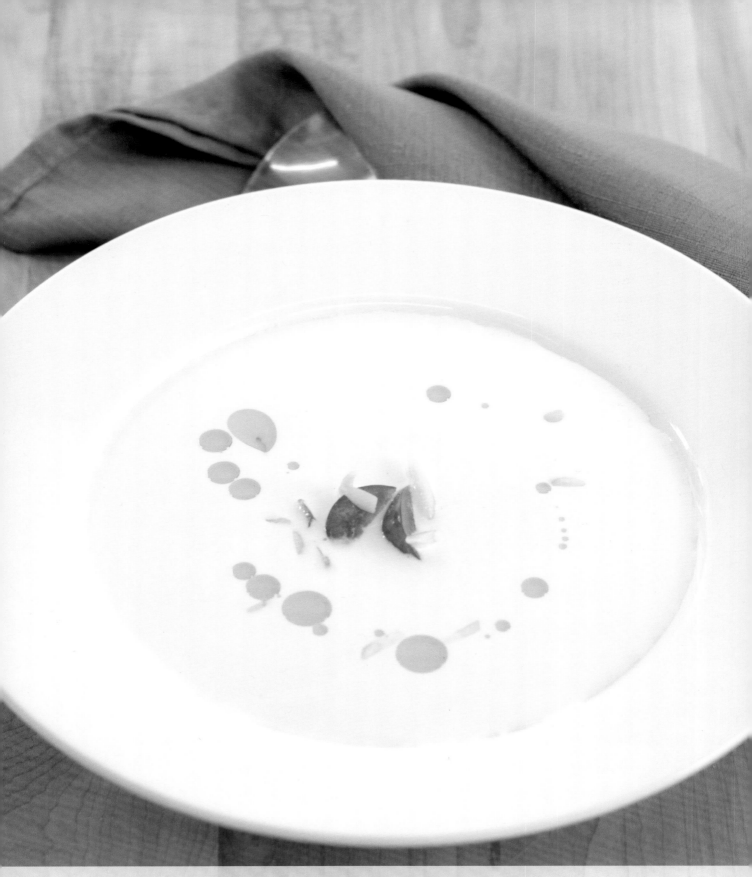

ALMOND & GARLIC GAZPACHO

Serves 6 | Ready in 6 hours

60g cashews, soaked 4 hours
150g almonds, toasted & ground
30 mL sherry
30 mL rice vinegar
120 mL camelina oil
10g (3 medium cloves) garlic
1 mL almond extract
7.5 mL salt
1.5 L water, boiled then cooled, to bring
    finished soup to 6 servings

300g grapes, quartered
30g slivered almonds, toasted
Alpha Balance™ Chili Oil to drizzle (see
    page 214)

This soup was a new flavour for our family, but it was an instant hit. It's a great soup for those hot summer evenings. It can be refrigerated for up to a week, and the grapes prepared as needed. – CG

PLACE soaked cashews in blender. Add ground almonds and enough water to blend. The mixture should resemble pancake batter. Add sherry, vinegar, almond extract, garlic, and salt. Slowly pour in camelina oil as mixture is blending. Add water a little bit at a time to keep mixture smooth.

POUR from blender into a bowl through fine sieve, using a spoon to press down on solids. Add enough water to make up 6 cups. Chill mixture for 1–3 hours.

TOAST slivered almonds. Pour soup into shallow bowls. Mound grapes in the centre of each bowl. Top with slivered almonds and drizzle with oil.

 TIP Cutting back on the grapes is an easy way to reduce the amount of carbs in this meal.

NET CARBS 15.3G   PROTEIN 8.5G PER SERVING

 GF   VEGAN   DAIRY FREE   VEG

BLACK BEAN SOUP with Cilantro Yogurt

Serves 6 | Ready in 45 minutes

75 mL of butter

100g celery, chopped

100g carrots, chopped

100g large sweet onion, chopped

15g (5 cloves) garlic, crushed

100g red bell pepper, chopped

5 mL chili powder

5 mL coriander

850g black beans, drained and rinsed

5 mL balsamic vinegar

1L vegetable broth

50 mL fresh lime juice

100g cherry tomatoes, sliced

250 mL Greek (10% mf) yogurt

50g fresh cilantro, chopped

Salt and pepper to taste

IN a large pot, sauté celery, carrots, and onion in butter until soft. Add garlic, red pepper, coriander, and chili powder. Season with salt and pepper.

ADD beans, balsamic vinegar and vegetable broth.

BRING to a boil and simmer for 15 minutes.

USING an immersion blender or a blender, blend until smooth but with some texture. Add lime juice.

IN a small bowl mix yogurt with cilantro. Pour soup into bowls. Top bowls with fresh tomatoes and cilantro yogurt.

NET CARBS 28G	PROTEIN 17.5G PER SERVING

GF   VEG

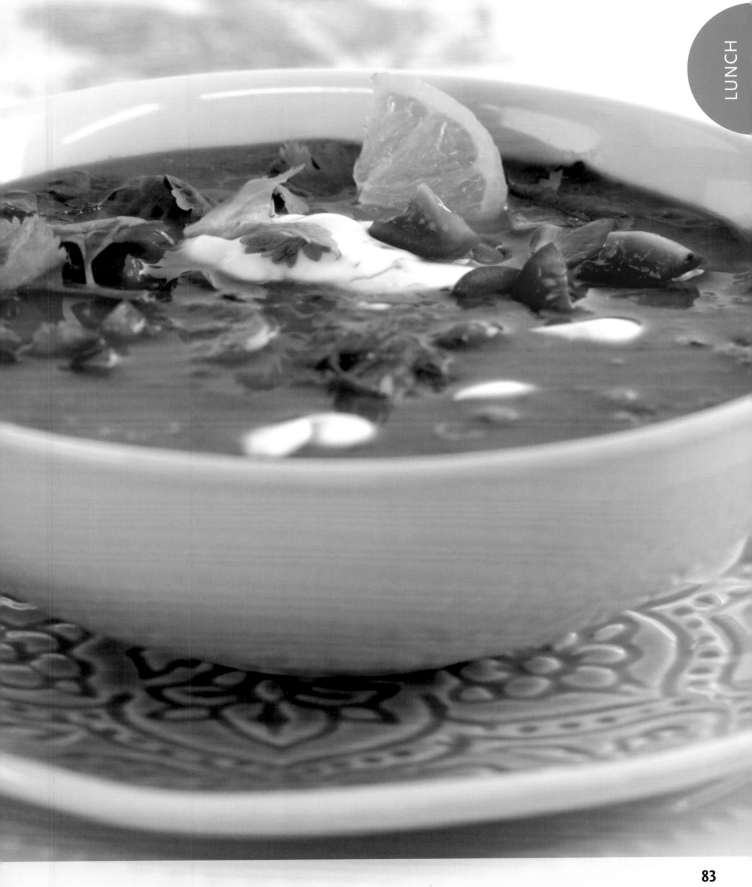

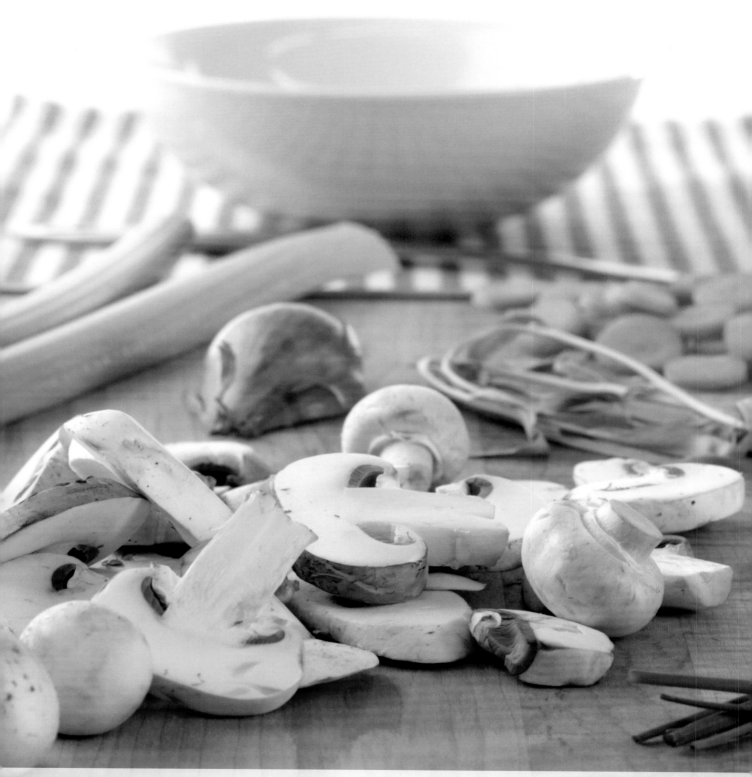

BUTTER MUSHROOM SOUP with Tarragon and Chives

Serves 4 | Ready in 30 minutes

60g butter
100g carrots, diced
100g celery stalks, diced
30g shallots, chopped
425g mushrooms, chopped
1L beef or vegetable broth
250 mL heavy (whipping) cream
10g chives, diced
3g tarragon, diced
Splash of white wine or sherry (optional)

MELT 30g of butter on medium heat in a large pot. Add celery, carrots, and shallots, and sauté until soft. Add mushrooms and let cook for about 3 minutes, until mushrooms brown and soften.

ADD broth and bring to a gentle boil, then reduce heat to low.

ADD remaining ingredients and purée.

 Serves nicely with crumbled bacon and blue cheese. Use a mix of white, brown, crimini and shiitake mushrooms.

NET CARBS 9.5G	PROTEIN 5.8G PER SERVING

 GF   VEG

85

BUTTER PANEER with Zucchini Rice

Serve 4 | Ready in 50 minutes

15g butter

15g onion, diced

9g fresh ginger, grated

9g (3 cloves) garlic, minced

15 mL coriander, dried

3 mL chili powder

45 mL tomato paste

5 mL fenugreek powder

15 mL garam masala or more to taste

5 mL sea salt

500 mL heavy (whipping) cream

250g Paneer cheese, cubed

Fresh cilantro sprigs for garnish

800g (4 medium) zucchini, pulsed in food processor until rice-like

Salt and pepper to taste

IN a medium sauce pan over low–medium heat, melt 10g of butter and add diced onion, ginger, garlic, and cook for two minutes or until soft and aromatic.

ADD dried spices to mixture and stir. Fold in tomato paste and cover pan, cook for 3 minutes.

REDUCE heat to low and add whipping cream and salt. Whisk.

ADD Paneer and keep warm.

IN a separate pan, over medium heat, melt 5g of butter and gently stir in zucchini until warm – about 5 minutes.

PLATE zucchini rice and top with Butter Paneer. Garnish with fresh cilantro.

 Make this recipe vegan by replacing the cheese with firm tofu, the butter with coconut oil, and the cream with coconut milk.

NET CARBS 13G	PROTEIN 14.6G PER SERVING

GF   VEG

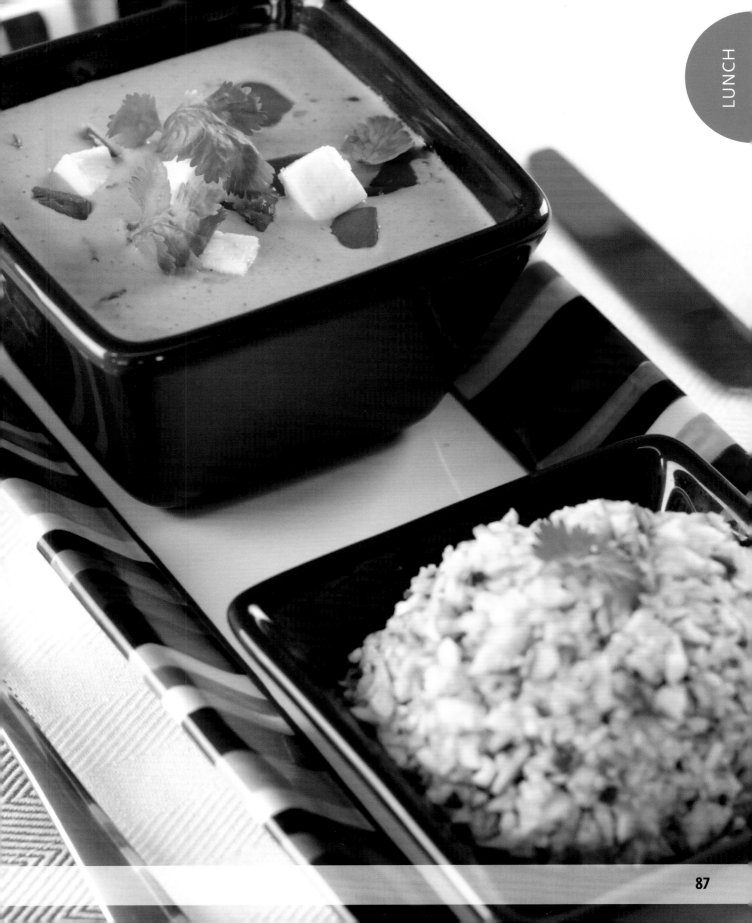

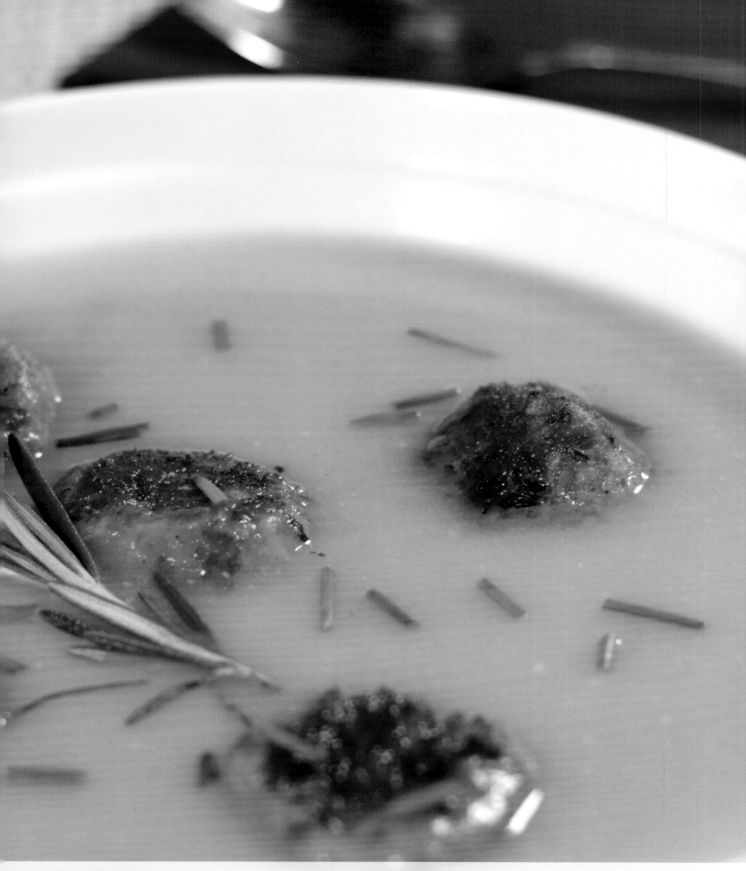

CELERIAC SOUP with Vegetarian Frikadelles

Serves 8 | Ready in 1 hour

SOUP

600g celeriac
500 mL vegetable stock
1500 mL water
30 mL Bragg's soy seasoning
Additional boiled water (optional)
Salt to taste
Green onions chopped for garnish

FRIKADELLES

65g glutinous rice (dry), rinsed and soaked
   overnight
250 mL vegetable stock
50g onions, minced
70g celery, minced
100g mushrooms, minced
70g cabbage, minced
100g carrot, grated fine
60g almonds, ground
50g coconut flour
300g pinto beans, cooked and mashed
15g garlic
5g fresh parsley, chopped fine
1g fresh rosemary, chopped fine
2g fresh oregano, chopped fine
1g fresh thyme, chopped fine
15 mL paprika
15 mL Bragg's soy seasoning
60g DME™ Coconut Oil for sautéing
30 mL red palm olein for frying
Salt to taste

Celeriac is a variety of celery that is prized for its large, edible root. The root should be brown and bumpy, but choose a celeriac that has no dark or soft spots. The shoots are edible as well and can be used in soups, stews and braises. —CG

SOUP

PEEL and cube celeriac. Add celeriac to stock and water, bring to boil, turn to simmer, and cook until celeriac is soft. Purée. Stir in Bragg's. Add water until desired thickness is reached. Salt to taste.

FRIKADELLES

DRAIN rice and put in pot with stock. Bring to boil, and immediately turn down to low simmer. Cook until all the water has been absorbed.

COOK beans until soft. Salt to taste. If the pot still contains water, simmer on low without lid until water is evaporated.

MINCE onions, celery, mushrooms, and cabbage in food processor in turn. Heat half the coconut oil in pan and brown onions together with celery. Add garlic, sauté until fragrant, and add to mixing bowl.

ADD remaining coconut oil to pan, and sauté mushrooms together with cabbage until mushrooms release their water. Salt to taste. Add to mixing bowl.

GRATE carrots fine. Grind almonds in nut grinder. Add both to mixing bowl.

ADD chopped herbs, paprika, cooked rice, and beans, then mash together until well combined. Stir in Bragg's. Mix in coconut flour so that mixture holds together well. Add more salt if necessary.

FORM balls from mixture and fry in pan to brown all sides. Add 5 frikadelles per bowl of soup, and garnish with green onions.

NET CARBS 21.5G	PROTEIN 8.4G PER SERVING

 GF VEGAN VEG

CHEESE FLATBREAD

Serves 4 | Ready in 35 minutes

50g almonds, finely ground

20g coconut flour

2g baking powder

60g Greek (10% mf) yogurt

1 egg

10g Parmesan cheese, grated fine

50g aged Cheddar, grated

10g garlic (3 cloves), minced (optional)

I modified this recipe from one developed by my sister, who has the baking skills in the family. I was so excited to have a low carb option that will serve the purpose of tasty sandwich slices. The Breakfast Flatbreads (page 22) are a non-cheesy variation. Leaving the garlic out makes it something you can have with a little jam at breakfast. — CG

PREHEAT oven to 175°C (350°F).

MIX dry ingredients in a bowl. Add yogurt, egg, and Cheddar and Parmesan. Stir until all ingredients are moist.

USING a parchment paper lined baking sheet, spread batter evenly about 1 cm thick and cut after baking, or form into 2-½ inch circles (or use a baking ring as a mold). Makes 8 rounds.

BAKE for 15–18 minutes.

 This is as good a place for a rant as any. Whatever you do in life, avoid non-fat dairy products. When you consume fat, it tells your body you're full. Non-fat dairy leaves you hungry, but fills you with empty carbohydrates (and calories) in the form of thickeners. No good can come of this. The higher the fat content, the better.

NET CARBS 2.3G	PROTEIN 10G PER SERVING, 2 ROUNDS EACH

GF   VEG

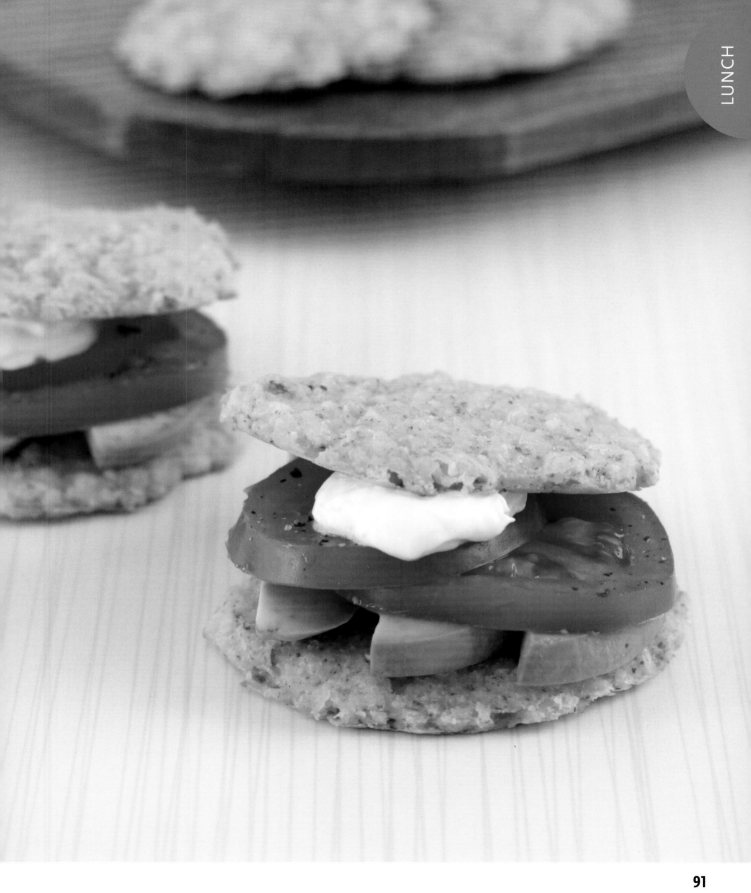

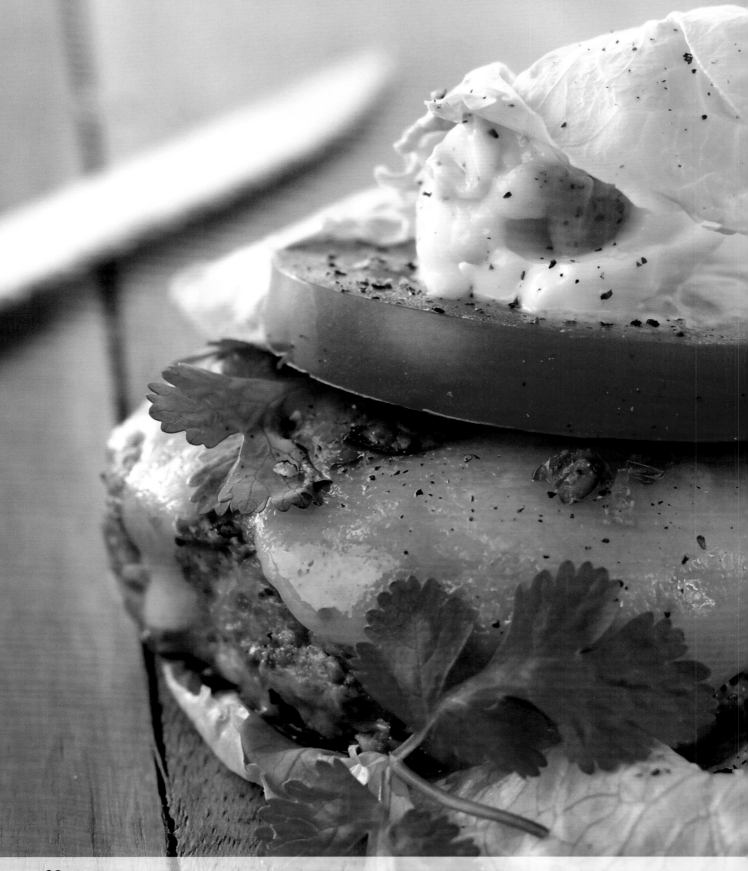

CILANTRO JALAPEÑO TURKEY BURGERS

Serves 4 | Ready in 25 minutes

500g ground turkey

3g fresh garlic, crushed or chopped

10g fresh cilantro, chopped

10g fresh jalapeño pepper, seeded, chopped

200g thick slices of strong white Cheddar, Havarti or Swiss

Salt and pepper to taste

4 large iceberg lettuce leaves, washed and dried

100g sliced tomato

30 mL Dijon mustard

30 mL Greek (10% mf) yogurt

Spicy, but not too spicy. These burgers hit the spot. Keep them in mind for family BBQs and moments when you just need a burger. —AT

IN a large bowl mix turkey, garlic, cilantro, and jalapeño until well incorporated.

FORM into four patties and cook in an oiled pan, or on barbeque, until fully cooked.

TOP burgers with cheese during the last few minutes of cooking; just enough to melt.

FOR plating, place lettuce with the burger patties on top.

TOP with mustard, yogurt, and tomato.

WRAP, and serve.

 Use gloves when handling the jalapeño, and avoid touching your eyes or mouth until your gloves are off. The extra step is worth the added flavour without any extra tears.

NET CARBS 8G	PROTEIN 40G PER SERVING

GF

COCONUT PRAWN BISQUE

Serves 6 | Ready in 1 hour

550g prawns (shell on)
60 mL red palm olein
2 whole star anise pods
60 mL dry sherry
1L fish or seafood stock
15 mL DME™ Coconut Oil
150g sliced leeks
15g (5 cloves) garlic, minced
Chili flakes to taste
Salt and pepper to taste
75 mL tomato paste
60 mL heavy (whipping) cream
Extra water or stock to thin if necessary
Alpha Balance™ Herbs de Provence Oil
    (page 214)
A few leaves of chopped parsley
Lemon wedges

This recipe is courtesy of Alpha Health Products and Chef Tom Liu. –CG

PEEL the prawns and reserve their shells. Roast the prawn shells over medium high heat in palm oil. Add star anise and continue to roast shells until fragrant. Deglaze with sherry and reduce by half. Scrape the sediment off the base of the pan and add stock. Simmer for 30 minutes to infuse the flavour. Strain and reserve.

IN a heavy pan, melt coconut oil and sauté leeks and garlic. Season with chili flakes and salt and pepper. Add tomato paste and cook for 3–5 minutes. Add prawns and cook. When cooked, remove prawns and reserve 1–2 per serving.

DEGLAZE the pan with the infused prawn stock. Purée whole mixture with heavy cream, thinning the soup with extra stock or water if necessary. Serve hot, with reserved prawns, a drizzle of Alpha Balance™ Herbs de Provence Oil (page 214), chopped parsley and some lemon wedges.

NET CARBS 8G	PROTEIN 23.3G PER SERVING

GF

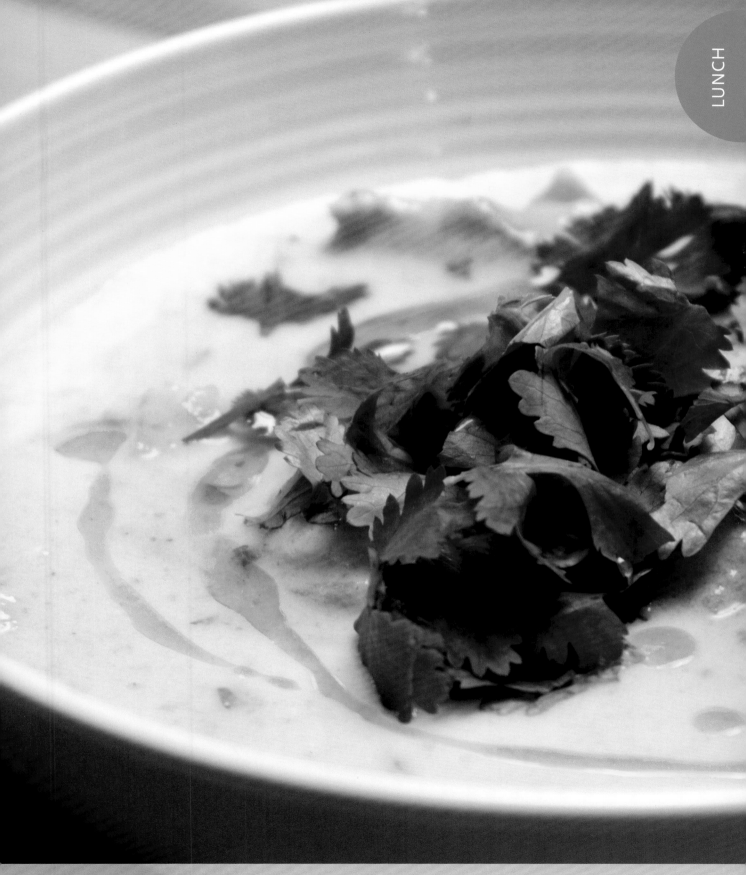

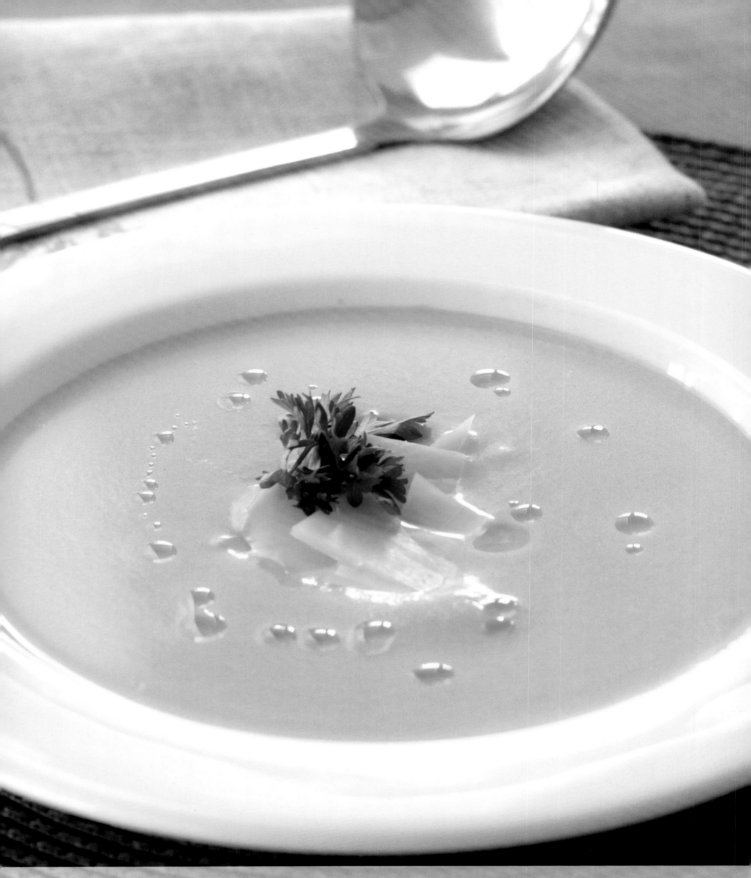

CREAM OF CARROT SOUP

Serves 8 | Ready in 40 minutes

15 mL Alpha Balance™ Oil

50g onion, diced fine

20g ginger, minced

400g carrots

15 mL maple syrup

250 mL vegetable stock

250 mL water

250 mL heavy (whipping) cream

Salt to taste

Pinch of cayenne pepper

We like the cream of carrot soup with crumbled feta and cracked black pepper. Strips of roasted bell pepper (char the skin to peel it off) are also a nice accompaniment. —CG

HEAT the oil in a pot over medium low. Sauté the onions until soft. Add the ginger and sauté until fragrant. Add the stock, water, carrots, and maple syrup. Bring to a boil. Turn the heat to medium and cook until the carrots are soft. Use an immersion blender to purée the soup. Add additional water to bring the soup to the desired consistency (it should coat the back of a spoon). Stir in the cream. Salt to taste. Add the pinch of cayenne.

 TIP The purée can be made ahead of time and frozen without the cream, which can be added at the point of reheating for a quick and easy meal.

NET CARBS 7.5G	PROTEIN 1.3G PER SERVING

GF   VEG

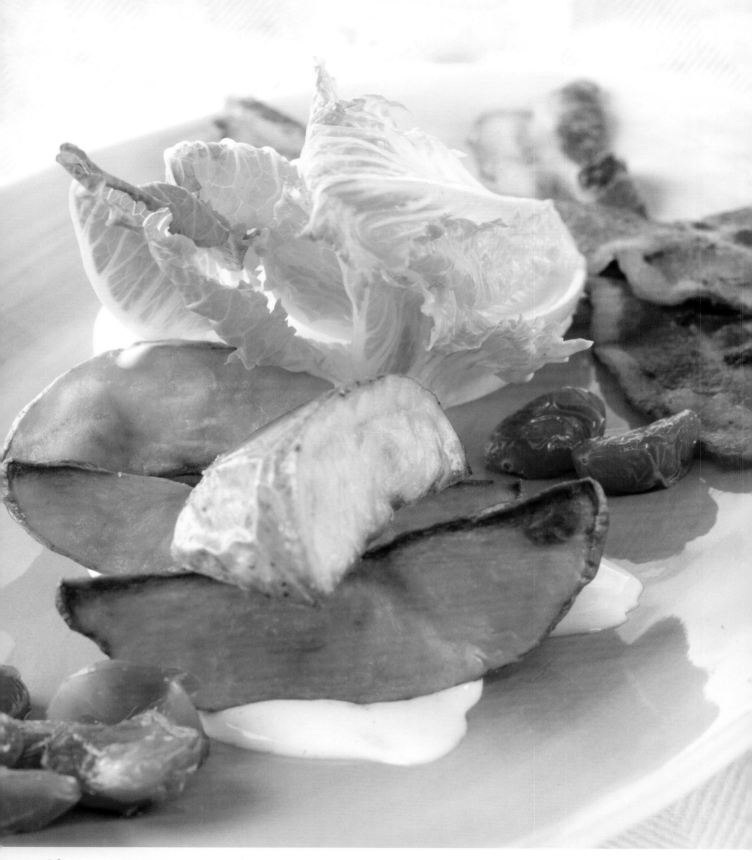

CRISPY BACON & POTATO WEDGE SALAD

with Grilled Romaine Lettuce & Roasted Tomato Mayonnaise

Serves 4 | Ready in 35 minutes

8 slices of cooked bacon, cooled and crumbled

450g (2 medium) potatoes cut into wedges

15 mL red palm oil

1.25 mL sea salt

1.25 mL fresh ground pepper

125g cherry tomatoes, seeded

125 mL mayonnaise

10 mL balsamic vinegar

2.5 mL Dijon mustard

4 romaine lettuce hearts, sliced in half

15 mL camelina oil

30 mL fresh lemon juice

COOK bacon until just crispy, and drain.

PREHEAT oven to 190°C (375°F). Toss potatoes in red palm oil, salt, and fresh ground pepper. Place skin side down on a lined baking sheet, and roast on the medium rack until crispy and golden, approximately 25 minutes.

LINE a cookie sheet with parchment paper, and place the cherry tomatoes in an even layer, flesh side down. Place in oven on the lower rack for last 15 minutes for cooking the potato wedges. Remove both and allow to cool on wire racks.

IN a small bowl, mix mayonnaise, balsamic vinegar, and Dijon mustard together, and then fold in roasted tomatoes.

ROLL romaine hearts in camelina oil and sprinkle with lemon juice.

GRILL on the barbeque for 1 minute each side, or in a grill pan on the stove top, until lightly charred and wilted.

PLATE the grilled romaine, potatoes and bacon on two plates, and drizzle with tomato mayo. Season to taste.

NET CARBS 26.8G	PROTEIN 9G PER SERVING

 GF DAIRY FREE

FETA SALAD with Strawberries and Toasted Almonds

Serves 4 | Ready in 15 minutes

120g sliced almonds

125 mL olive oil

60 mL apple cider vinegar

5 mL Bragg's soy seasoning

5 mL Dijon mustard

15g (1 small) shallot, chopped

250g (1 head) butter lettuce, washed, dried,
    torn into bite-size pieces

700g (1 head) romaine lettuce, washed,
    dried, torn into bite-size pieces

100g (2) endives, washed, dried, rough
    chopped

200g sheep feta, crumbled

150g strawberries, sliced

IN a dry skillet, toast the almonds over medium heat until just browned.

REMOVE from heat and cool.

IN a blender, or with a whisk, blend oil, vinegar, Dijon mustard, Bragg's and shallot. Set aside.

IN a large bowl, toss the lettuce, endive, feta and strawberries.

ADD dressing ten minutes before serving so the flavours have a chance to get to know each other. Top with almonds just before plating.

NET CARBS 10.5G   PROTEIN 16.9G PER SERVING

GF   VEG

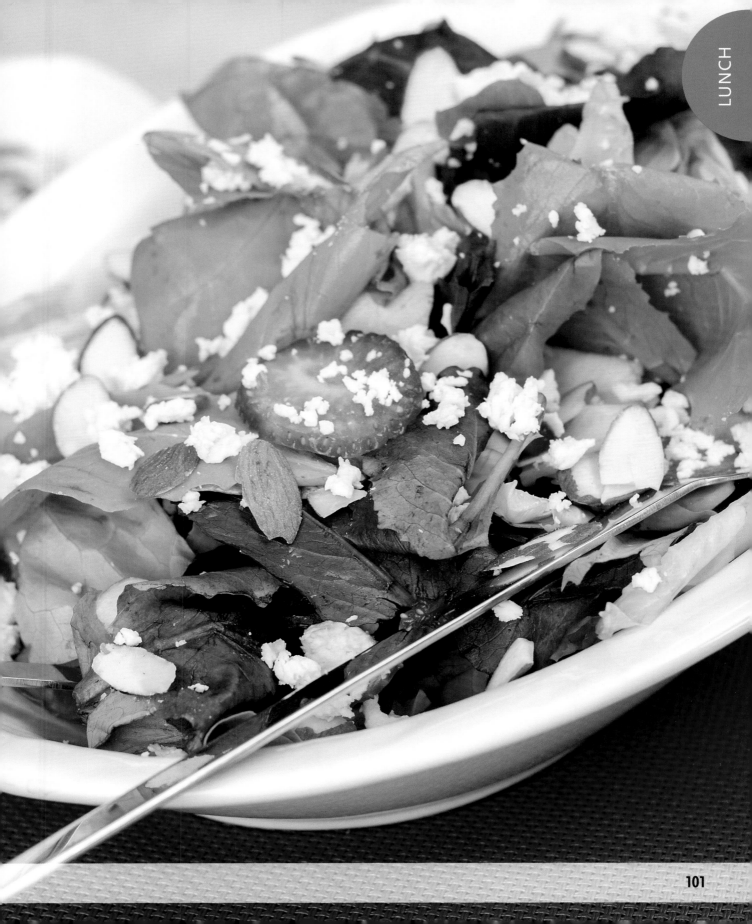

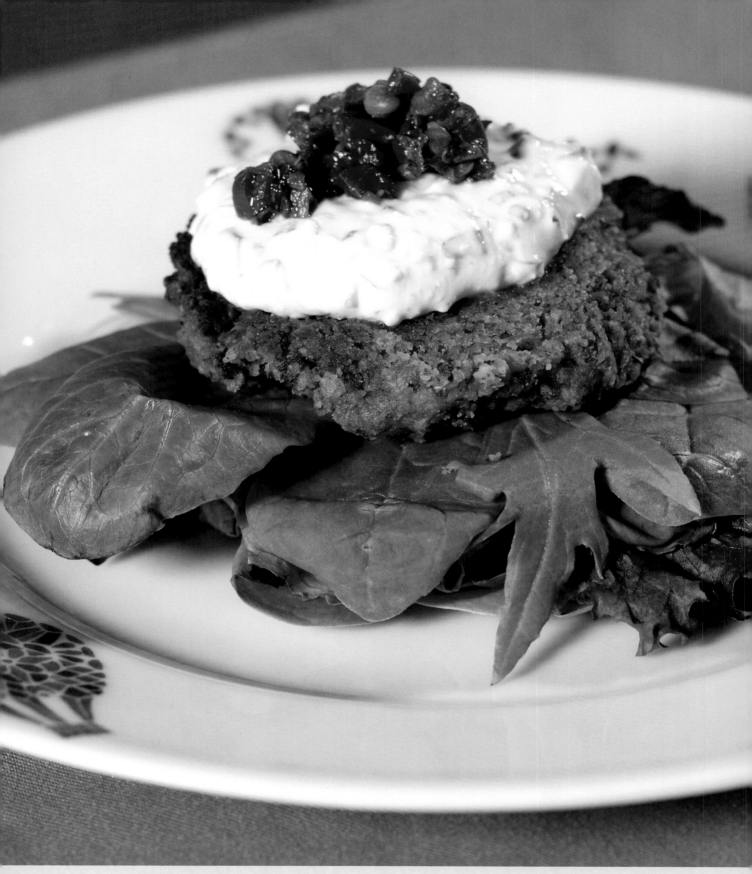

HAZELNUT SQUASH FRITTERS

Serves 6 | Ready in 35 minutes

FRITTERS

300g Hazelnut Squash Dessert (page 205)

10g (3 cloves) garlic, roasted
20g flaxseed, fresh ground
100g hazelnuts, ground
15 mL red palm olein for frying

OLIVE TAPENADE

100g olives, pitted
10g (3 cloves) garlic
16g capers
30 mL Alpha Balance™ Oil

240g mixed greens

Use the basic recipe for Hazelnut Squash Dessert (page 205).
– CG

FRITTERS

ADD roasted garlic to the purée, along with ground flaxseed and ground hazelnuts. The mixture should hold a ball shape when formed, and will still be sticky. Form 12 balls and set them aside on parchment paper.

HEAT palm olein in a non-stick pan over medium heat. When hot, press the balls into fritters, shake the pan to spread out the oil, place the fritters in the pan. Do not crowd. Let brown on one side, about two minutes, then flip and brown the other side.

SERVE over a bed of mixed greens with the olive tapenade and Herbed Feta Sour Cream (page 217).

DIVIDE into 12 or more portions for a smaller, appetizer size.

FINISHED fritters can be refrigerated or frozen, and reheated in the oven as necessary.

TAPENADE

MINCE the garlic. Chop the olives and capers on a cutting board. Combine the ingredients in a mixing bowl with the oil. Let stand for 15 minutes to meld flavours. Serve as garnish. May be refrigerated for up to two weeks.

 The mixed greens may be dressed (try the Gursche House Dressing on page 216) or undressed, depending on your preference. You can also play with the spices a bit. Add some cumin for a North African flavour. Or mix in some sweet herbs, like basil or cilantro. If you're using a partial portion of purée, adjust the hazelnuts and flax as needed.

NET CARBS 8.8G	PROTEIN 2.9G PER SERVING

 GF   VEGAN   DAIRY FREE   VEG

LASAGNA SALAD

Serves 2 | Ready in 20 minutes

SALAD

200g zucchini, sliced or use a carrot peeler
   to make thin ribbons
200g fresh buffalo Mozzarella, sliced
50g of basil leaves, sliced into ribbons
100g of sliced Roma tomatoes

DRESSING

30 mL balsamic vinegar
45 mL Alpha Balance™ Oil
3g (1 small clove) garlic
Salt and pepper

This low carb salad will satisfy a lasagna craving! —AT

WHISK dressing ingredients together in a bowl and let sit, stirring again just before serving.

ON two plates, begin layering zucchini, cheese, basil, and tomato. After the first round of layers are complete, drizzle 5 mL of dressing over the layer.

MAKE one more layer, and drizzle another spoon of dressing over the lasagna and serve.

NET CARBS 9.1G	PROTEIN 24.5G PER SERVING

GF   VEG

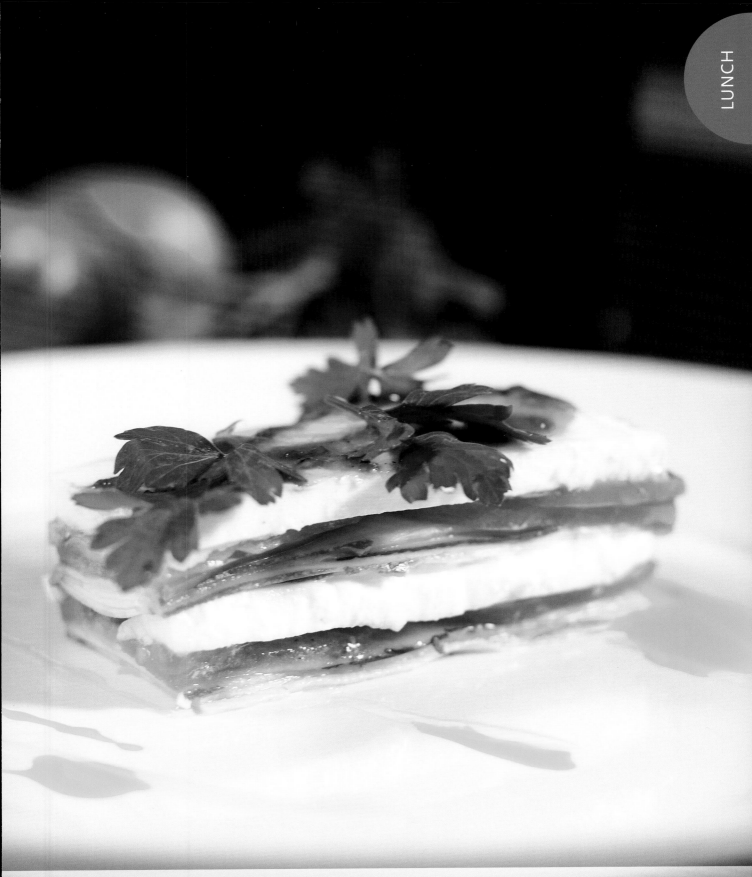

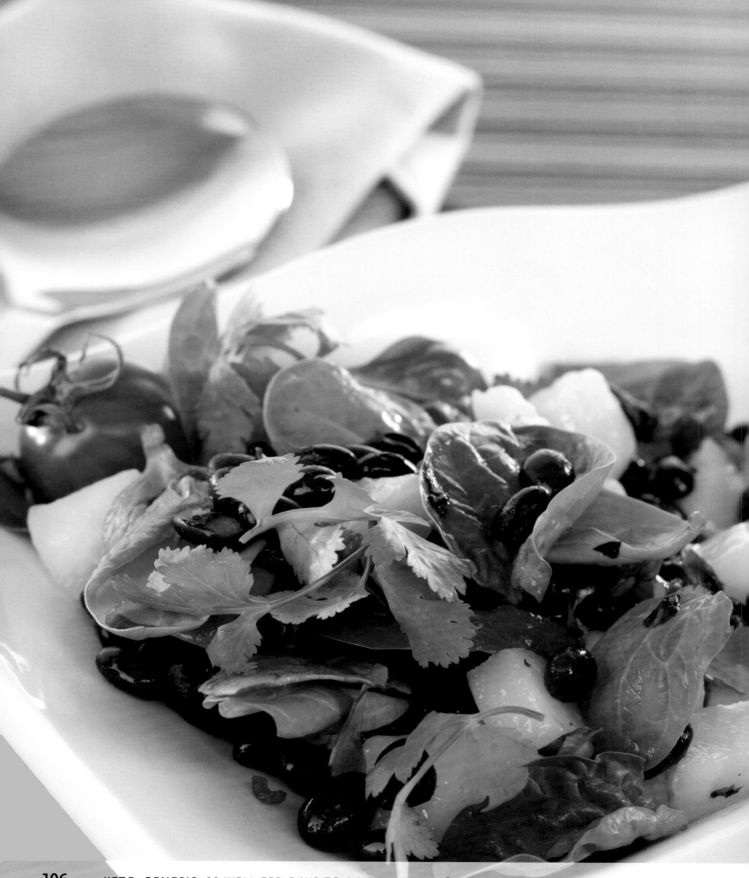

MANGO AND BLACK BEAN SALAD

Serves 4 | Ready in 15 minutes

DRESSING

30 mL apple cider vinegar
15 mL olive oil
5 mL roasted sesame oil
3g (1 clove) garlic, crushed
Pinch of crushed red pepper flakes
Salt and pepper

SALAD

420g canned black beans, rinsed and
    drained
200g fresh ripe mango, peeled and diced
100g baby spinach, washed and dried
50g green onion, diced
50g Thai basil, rinsed and chopped

BLEND dressing ingredients in a food processor or blender, or whisk for a few seconds.

COMBINE salad ingredients.

POUR dressing over salad and toss.

NET CARBS 18.5G	PROTEIN 7.6G PER SERVING

 GF VEGAN DAIRY FREE VEG

MARINATED EGGPLANT & SMOKED MOZZA STACKS

Serves 4 | Ready in 55 minutes

800g eggplant, sliced into 8 equal rounds

Sea salt (about 15 mL)

15 mL balsamic vinegar

5 mL fresh lemon juice

5 mL maple syrup

150 mL olive oil

400g smoked Mozzarella, shredded

200g Roma tomatoes, sliced thin

50g pitted green olives, chopped

50g fresh basil

5g fresh thyme

2.5g fresh oregano

Fresh ground pepper and sea salt to taste

PREHEAT oven to 190°C (375°F).

SPRINKLE eggplant with sea salt and let stand for 15 minutes, rinse and pat dry.

IN a large non-metallic bowl, toss eggplant with vinegar, lemon juice, maple syrup and olive oil. Save remaining marinade for plating.

IN a large baking dish, lay the eggplant flat and bake for 15–20 minutes, turning halfway, until soft. Remove from oven.

TOP with a layer of cheese and sliced tomato, and return to oven for 2 minutes, so cheese is just melted.

PLATE two eggplant stacks per plate, one on top of the other. Sprinkle with fresh herbs and olives.

DRIZZLE with remaining dressing.

SEASON and serve.

 Use hummus or Walnut Hummus (page 136) instead of cheese to make this a vegan dish.

NET CARBS 9.8G	PROTEIN 25G PER SERVING

GF   VEG

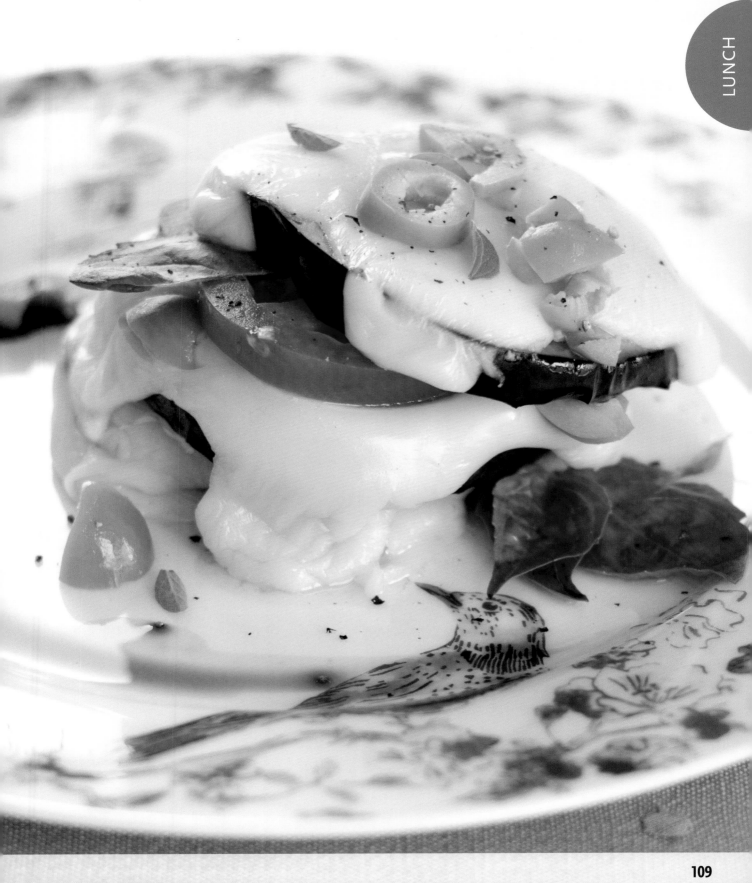

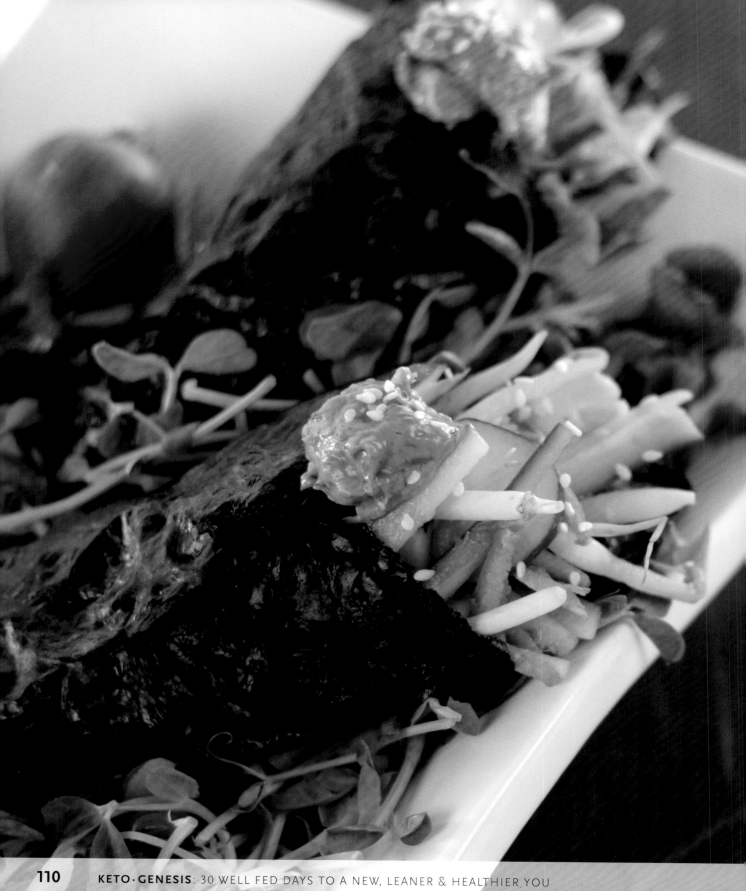

NORI SALAD WRAP with Peanut Sauce

Serves 2 | Ready in 20 minutes

SAUCE

15 mL natural, no sugar added peanut butter
15 mL lime juice
5g fresh cilantro
5 mL tamari or soy sauce alternative
5 mL honey or maple syrup

FILLING

100g cucumber, cut into matchsticks
100g red radish, sliced
200g (1 large) avocado, cubed
50g carrot, shredded
50g bean sprouts or pea shoots

4 sheets of nori

Satisfy any sushi craving with this quick recipe. —AT

COMBINE all sauce ingredients in a blender.

IN a large bowl, combine filling ingredients.

LAY nori sheets flat on a dish diagonally, pile filling into center, and drizzle sauce over vegetables.

FOLD bottom corner of nori to secure filling, fold over, and eat!

NET CARBS 13.5G	PROTEIN 8G PER SERVING

 GF   VEGAN   DAIRY FREE VEG

NOT YOUR MOTHER'S POTATO SALAD

Serves 2 | Ready in 30 minutes

500g cauliflower, steamed and cooled,
   chopped into bite-size pieces
2 hardboiled eggs, cooled and diced
200g celery, washed and diced
50g red onions, chopped
125 mL Greek (10% mf) yogurt
15 mL yellow or Dijon mustard
15 mL apple cider vinegar
15g fresh dill, chopped

The humble cauliflower steps in to make this familiar favourite a low carb meal! – AT

SOAK onions in cold water for 5 minutes, then drain. This gives onions a more mild flavour.

TOSS all ingredients together and refrigerate for one hour before serving.

SEASON with pepper but reserve seasoning with salt until serving.

 Boil eggs the night before, making this salad a time saver. Keep in mind that any recipe in this book longs for the addition of more vegetables; so if your carbs are looking good for today, add more greens please!

NET CARBS 13.8G	PROTEIN 19.5G PER SERVING

GF   VEG

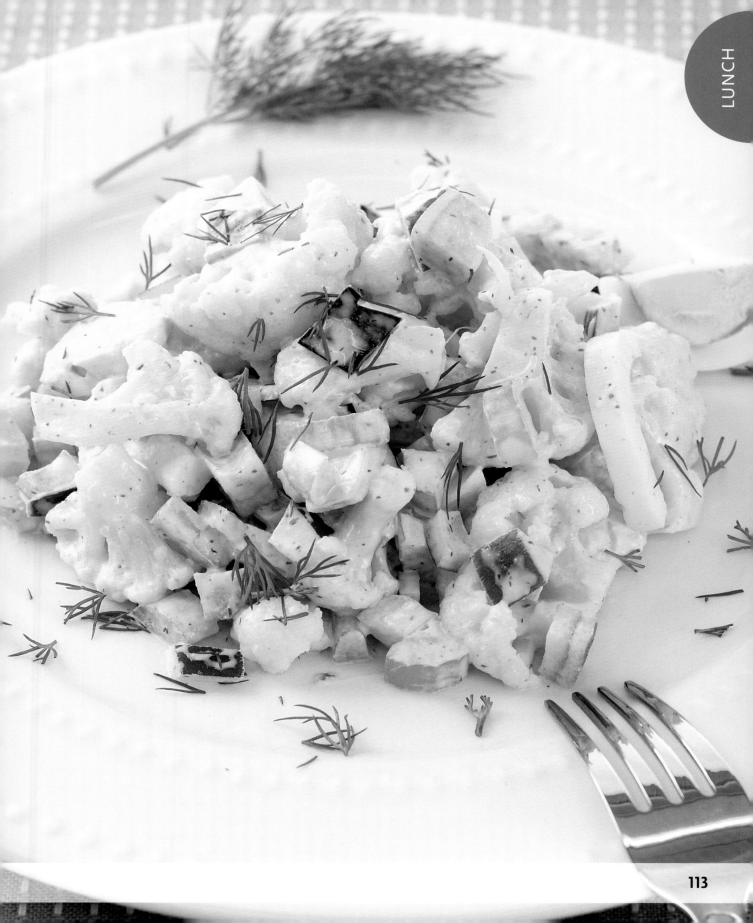

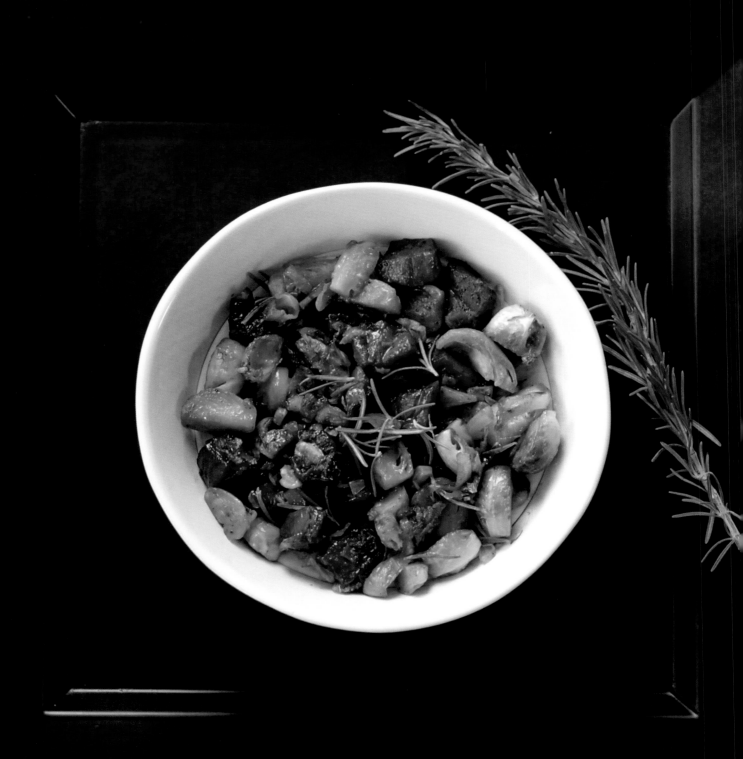

PAN FRIED BRUSSELS SPROUTS with Pancetta

Serves 2 | Ready in 20 minutes

30g butter

6g (2 small cloves) garlic, chopped

200g Brussels sprouts, washed and
    quartered

100g pancetta, cubed

15 mL balsamic vinegar

5 mL maple syrup

5 mL Dijon mustard

5g fresh rosemary, chopped

*When people say they don't like Brussels sprouts, they almost always mean they don't like steamed, bland mini cabbages. Change their minds with these crispy, buttery bites. Mmmmm.
– AT*

MELT butter in a large cast iron pan on medium heat. Add garlic and sauté until fragrant. Add Brussels sprouts and sauté until soft, about ten minutes. Add balsamic vinegar, maple syrup, Dijon mustard, and rosemary, stirring constantly.

WHEN Brussels sprouts start to get crispy, fold in pancetta and cook for 1 minute.

REMOVE and serve.

NET CARBS 9.3G	PROTEIN 13G PER SERVING

GF

PEAR & PROSCIUTTO ARUGULA SALAD

with Fresh Lemon Dressing

Serves 2 | Ready in 15 minutes

120 mL olive oil

90 mL fresh lemon juice

5 mL raw honey

2.5 mL sea salt

2.5 mL fresh ground black pepper

75g baby arugula

30g baby spinach

25g fresh basil leaves

100g fresh pear, chopped

100g Italian prosciutto, chopped

100g soft goat cheese

Salt and pepper to taste

BLEND or whisk olive oil, lemon juice, honey, salt, and pepper until emulsified.

TOSS the arugula, spinach, basil, pears, and prosciutto with dressing in a separate bowl.

TOP with crumbled goat cheese and lots of pepper and serve immediately.

 If prepping salad ahead of time, toss the sliced pears in lemon juice to prevent them from turning brown.

NET CARBS 18G	PROTEIN 23G PER SERVING

GF

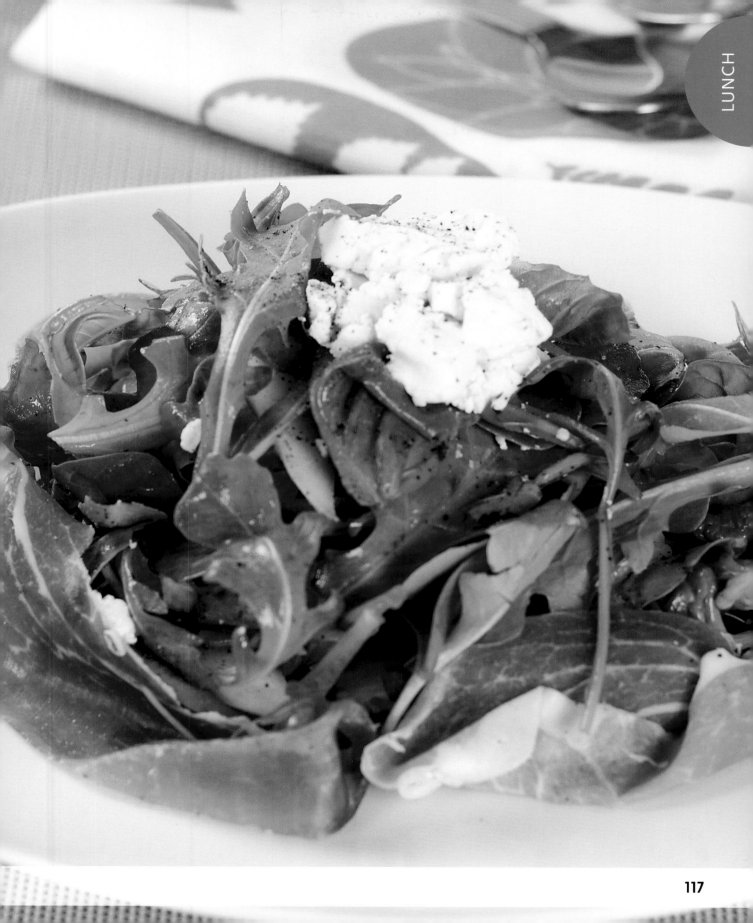

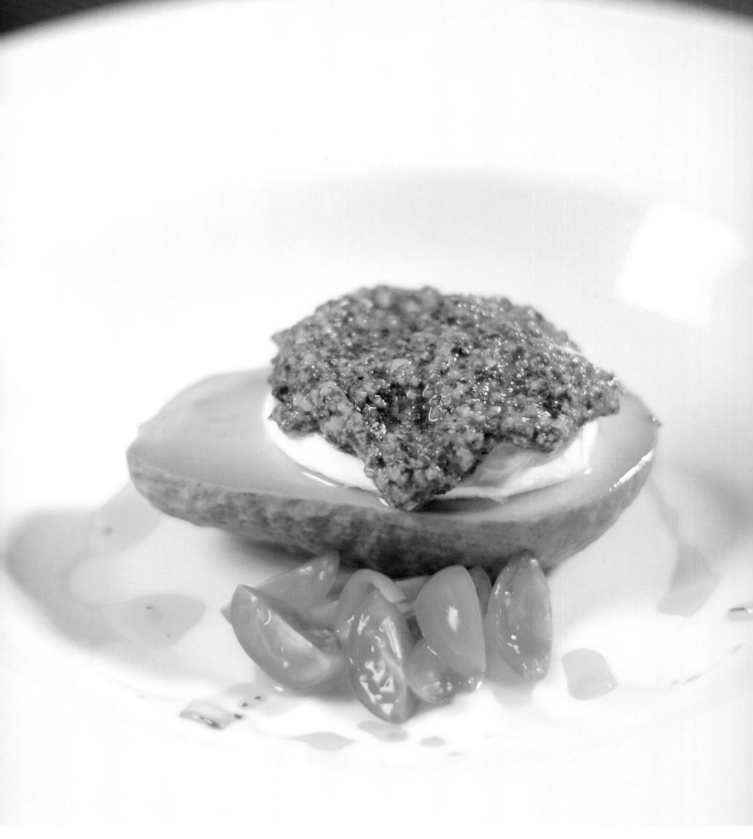

POACHED EGG STUFFED AVOCADO with Lemon & Herb Pesto

Serves 1 or 2 | Ready in 20 minutes

PESTO

45 mL Alpha Balance™ Oil
50g fresh basil leaves
50g fresh baby spinach leaves
15 mL lemon juice
3g (1 small clove) garlic
1 pinch each of salt and pepper

200g avocado, halved with pit removed
2 eggs, poached

100g cherry tomatoes, chopped

IN a food processor, pulse pesto ingredients until smooth.

POACH eggs until soft, or medium soft.

PLACE the eggs gently into the hollow of each avocado.

TOP with pesto and tomatoes.

NET CARBS 10G	PROTEIN 20G PER SERVING

 GF　 DAIRY FREE　VEG

POACHED HALIBUT

Serves 2 | Ready in 20 minutes

1 L fish or chicken broth

100 mL fresh lemon juice

3g (3 sprigs) fresh rosemary

5g (5 sprigs) fresh thyme

6g (2 cloves) garlic, diced

15 mL olive oil

7 mL fresh ground pepper

7 mL coarse sea salt

340g (2 steaks) halibut, skin removed,
   rinsed and patted dry

10g fresh chives, chopped

2 lemon wedges

This simple meal pairs well with Cauliflower Mash (page 148).
– AT

IN a large skillet, bring the broth, garlic, lemon juice, rosemary, and thyme to a slow boil.

RUB the halibut steaks with olive oil, pepper, and sea salt.

GENTLY place the halibut steaks in the broth. Turn off heat and cover. Cook until the flesh is firm and opaque, about 8 minutes.

REMOVE halibut and return the broth to a boil.

POUR broth into 2 deep bowls and add halibut steaks, garnish with fresh chives and fresh lemon wedges and serve.

 You can substitute the halibut for salmon or tilapia.

NET CARBS 7.7G	PROTEIN 28G PER SERVING

 GF   DAIRY FREE

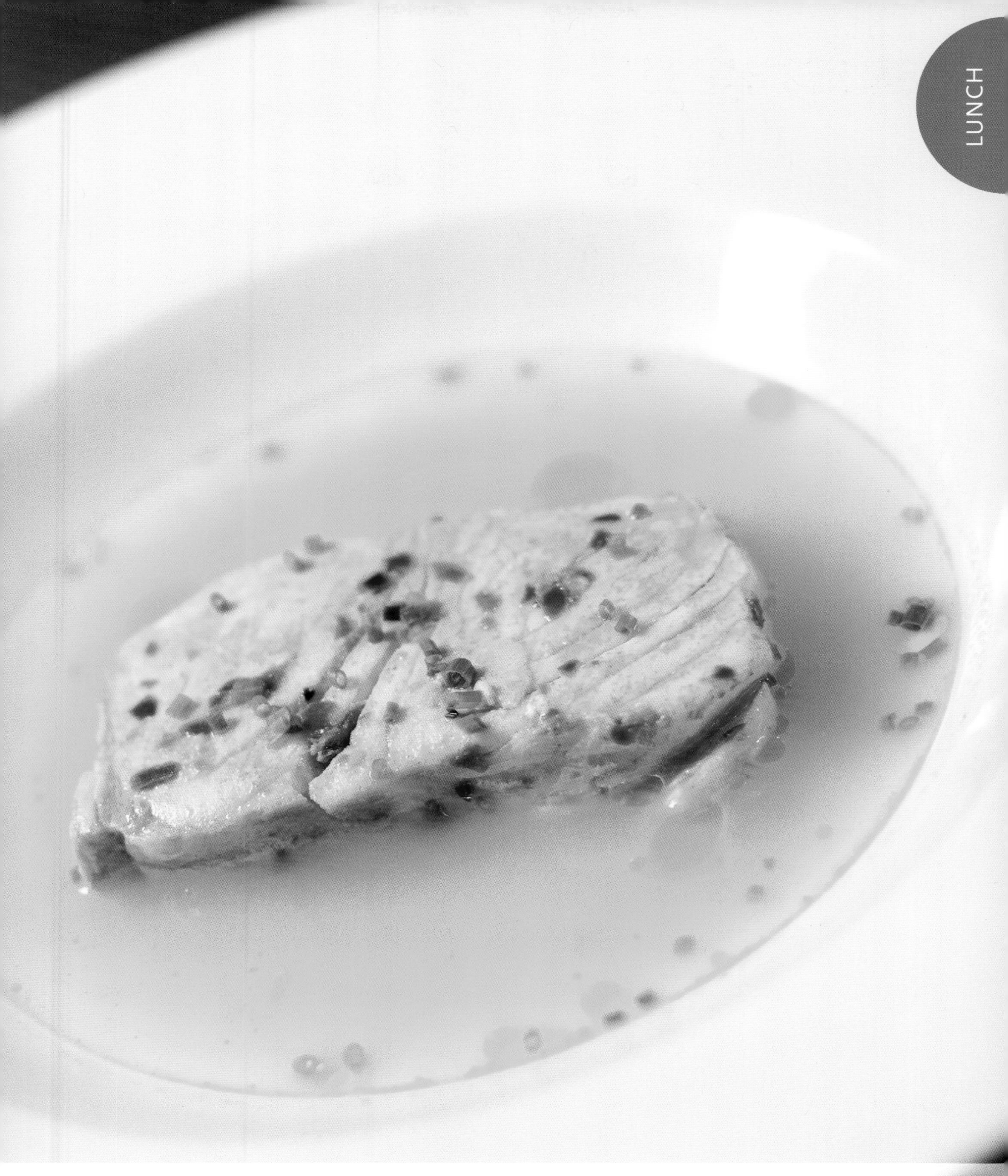

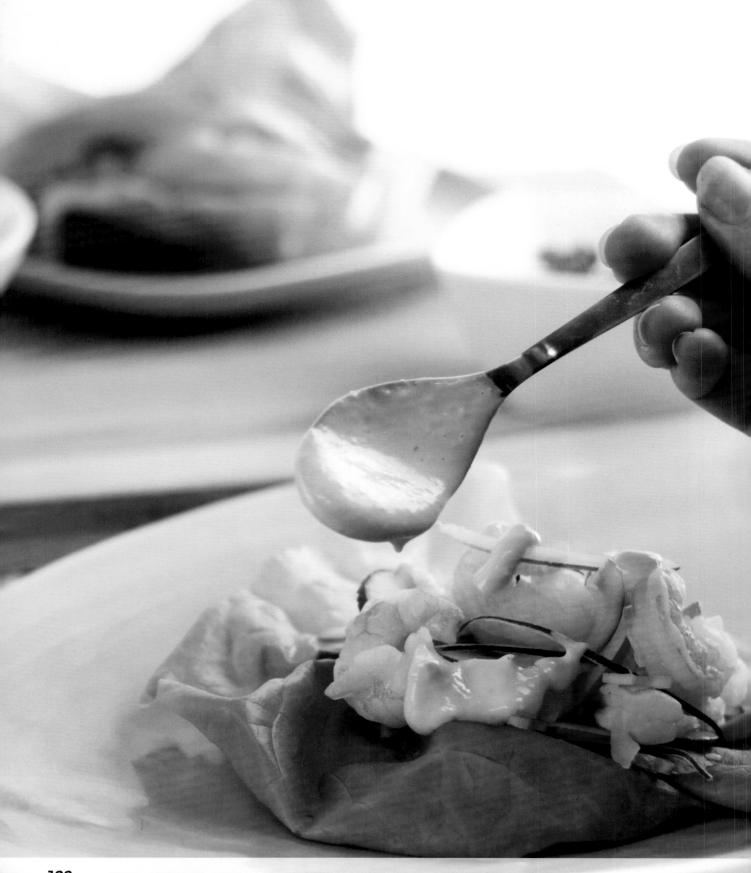

PRAWN COCKTAIL BUTTER LETTUCE WRAPS

Serves 4 | Ready in 25 minutes

PRAWNS

400g cooked shelled prawns, chilled
100g daikon or red radish, chopped
25g red onion, chopped
50g celery, diced
100g butter lettuce, washed and dried
10 mL lemon juice

COCKTAIL SAUCE

15 mL plain yogurt
5 mL horseradish, grated
5 mL ketchup
5 mL lemon juice
Dash of Tabasco sauce

This recipe was devoured immediately after it was photographed. — AT

IN a bowl, gently toss prawns, radish, onion, celery, and lemon juice. Season with salt and pepper.

MIX cocktail sauce ingredients together and set aside.

SERVE family style, with a bowl of washed lettuce leaves, a bowl of sauce, and the prawns, to be assembled into wraps.

 Use pre-cooked frozen prawns and thaw as needed for the recipe.

NET CARBS 4G	PROTEIN 20.8G PER SERVING

GF

RAINBOW CABBAGE SALAD with Toasted Sesame and Miso Dressing

Serves 4 (or 6 as a side salad) | Ready in 20 minutes

100g green cabbage, shredded
100g red cabbage, shredded
100g savoy cabbage, shredded
50g red bell pepper, diced
50g orange bell pepper, diced
50g yellow bell pepper, diced
50g grape or cherry tomatoes, sliced
100g green onion, sliced
75g Thai basil or cilantro
30 mL light miso paste
75 mL Alpha Balance™ Oil
5 mL roasted sesame oil
5 mL Dijon mustard
30 mL fresh lime juice
Dash of Tabasco sauce
Salt and pepper to taste
25g toasted black and white sesame seeds

Dig into this fresh salad for lunch, or pair with fish for dinner.
– AT

PLACE all vegetables and coriander in a large bowl and toss.

IN a blender or with a whisk, blend miso, Alpha Balance™ Oil, sesame oil, mustard, lime juice and Tabasco.

POUR dressing over salad, and toss. Refrigerate for one hour before serving. Add sesame seeds just before plating.

NET CARBS 9.4G		PROTEIN 4.8G PER SERVING	

 GF   VEGAN   DAIRY FREE   VEG

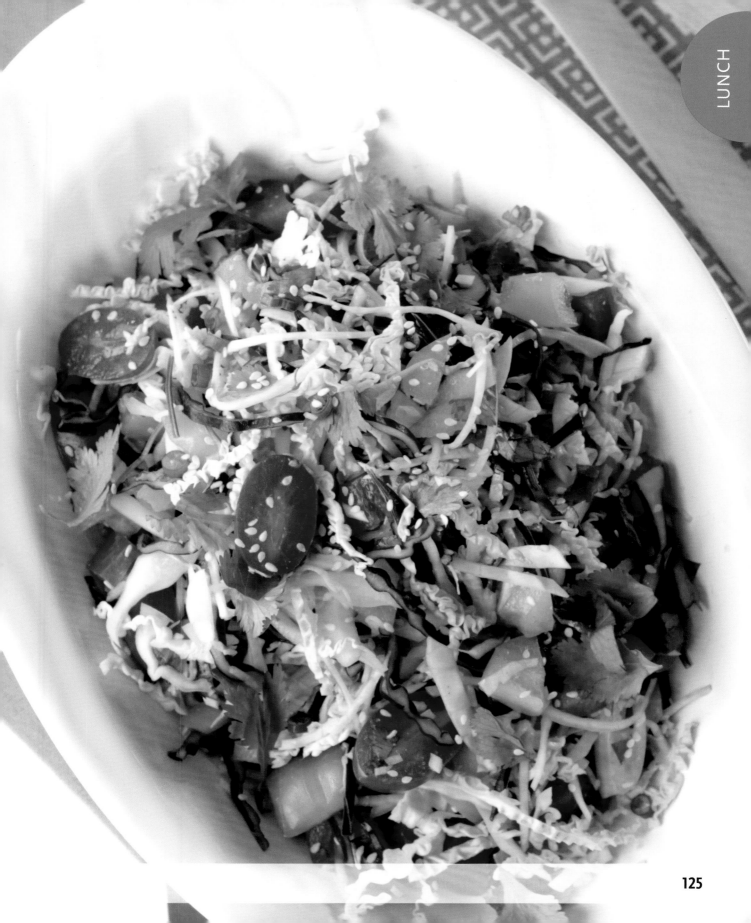

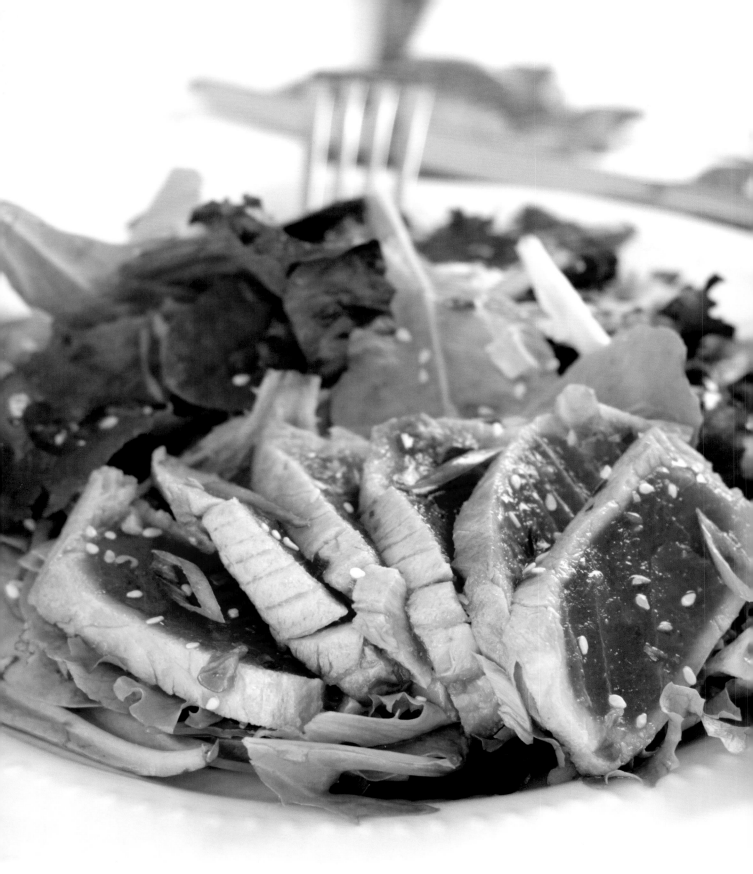

SEARED TUNA with Lime Vinaigrette

Serves 4 | Ready in 20 minutes

400g tuna steaks, 3 cm or thicker

45 mL Alpha Balance™ Oil

2.5g (1 small) Thai chili, minced

5g garlic, minced

10g ginger, sliced to thin matchsticks

10g scallion greens, sliced thin

7.5 mL lime zest

2g coconut sugar

45 mL Bragg's soy seasoning

30 mL lime juice

30 mL DME™ Coconut Oil

10g ginger, sliced thin (for frying)

Pinch of salt

200g mixed salad greens

This is a quick, light meal with lots of flavour. If you really like it spicy, double up on the Thai chili. Cut the portion sizes in half for eight quick appetizers. —CG

DRY the tuna with paper towels, and set aside.

POUR Alpha Balance™ Oil into a small bowl. Mince the chili, garlic, and ginger, and add to the oil. Chop the scallion greens fine, zest the lime, and add both to the oil.

DISSOLVE the sugar into the Bragg's soy sauce. Add to the oil. Add the lime juice, and blend with a fork.

MELT the coconut oil in a heavy pan over medium high heat. Slice the remaining ginger thin. When the oil shimmers, add the ginger. Salt the tuna lightly. When the ginger becomes fragrant, move it to the side of the pan, and place the tuna steaks in the pan. Sear on all sides for about two minutes each, or until the tuna browns lightly.

REMOVE and set aside to rest.

DIVIDE the salad greens onto four plates. Slice the tuna thin, and arrange evenly on the four plates. Drizzle lettuce and tuna with 2–3 tablespoons of vinaigrette per plate. Serve.

NET CARBS 3.5G	PROTEIN 26.5G PER SERVING

 GF

 DAIRY FREE

SMOKED SALMON TARTAR in Endive Cups

Serves 2 (or 4 as an appetizer) | Ready in 30 minutes

200g smoked salmon filet, chopped

100g cucumber, diced

50g green onion, diced

5g fresh dill

5 mL grainy Dijon mustard

5g capers, drained

15 mL olive oil

Salt and pepper

200g endive, washed and patted dry,
    for serving

This recipe would work well with any smoked fish, and would be very nice with tuna sashimi. — AT

GENTLY combine all ingredients and let marinate for 20 minutes.

FILL endive leaves with filling and serve.

 Pulse all ingredients except endive in a food processor to make a lovely paté for sliced cucumber topped with goat cheese.

NET CARBS 3.2G   PROTEIN 20.6G PER SERVING

 GF   DAIRY FREE

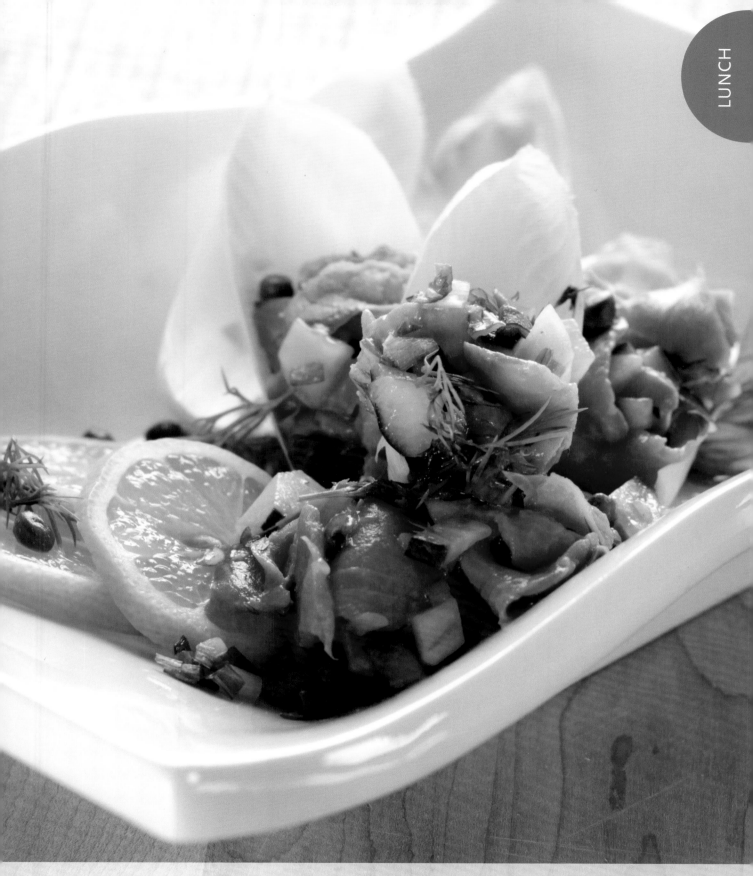

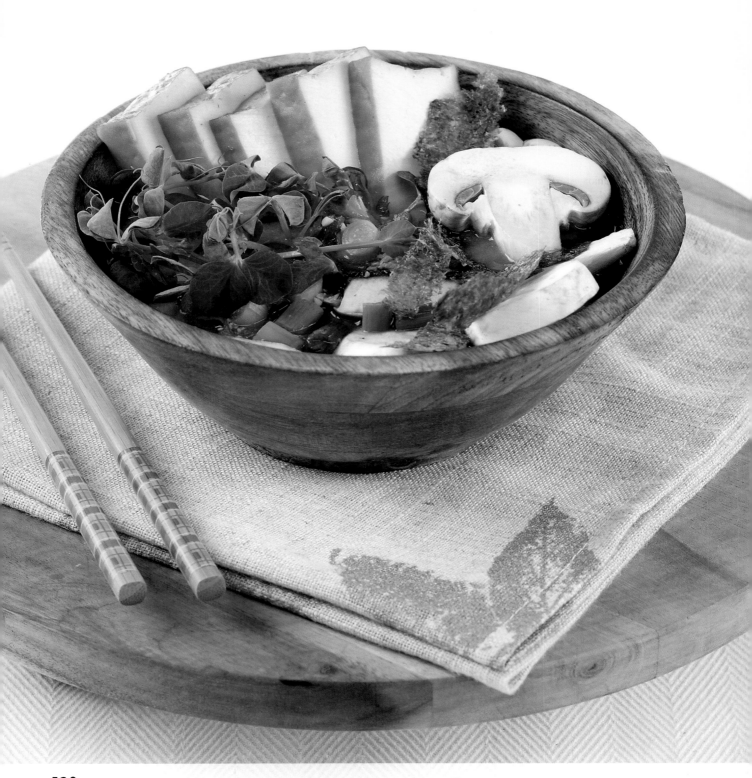

SMOKED TOFU MISO SOUP

Serves 2 | Ready in 15 minutes

100g miso paste

1L vegetable broth

5 mL garlic chili paste

100g fresh mushrooms, sliced

50g smoked tofu

100g fresh pea shoots

50g green onion, chopped

1 sheet roasted nori, crumbled

This soup is fast and looks beautiful. A perfect soup for vegetarians and omnivores alike. — AT

HEAT broth until steaming. Add miso paste and whisk until fully incorporated.

ADD garlic chili paste and mushrooms. Cook for 4 minutes, and remove from heat.

IN two soup bowls, put equal amounts of tofu, pea shoots and green onion and pour 250 mL of broth into each bowl.

TOP with crumbled nori flakes and serve.

TIP Any tofu will work, or add more vegetables and omit the tofu if you would like a soy-free option.

NET CARBS 19.7G	PROTEIN 12.5G PER SERVING

 GF   VEGAN   DAIRY FREE VEG

SWEET & SALTY BROCCOLI SALAD

with Crispy Bacon and Red Grapes

Serves 3 for Lunch (or 4 as a side dish) | Ready in 40 minutes

500g broccoli crowns, cut into
   bite-size pieces
125g seedless red grapes, slice in half
125g pumpkin seeds, gently roasted
10 slices of bacon
125 mL Greek (10% mf) yogurt
50g red onion, diced
30 mL balsamic vinegar
Salt and pepper to taste

IN a large frying pan cook the bacon over medium high heat, turning for even cooking. Remove when cooked and getting crispy. Drain on paper towel. When cooled, crumble and set aside.

TOAST pumpkin seeds on low heat for 5–10 minutes, remove from heat and cool.

IN a large bowl, combine the grapes, broccoli, and onion, tossing gently until well mixed.

IN a small bowl, add yogurt and balsamic vinegar, and whisk until uniform.

TOSS broccoli mix with dressing, fold in bacon and pumpkin seeds, season, and serve.

NET CARBS 20.7G	PROTEIN 34.5G PER SERVING

GF

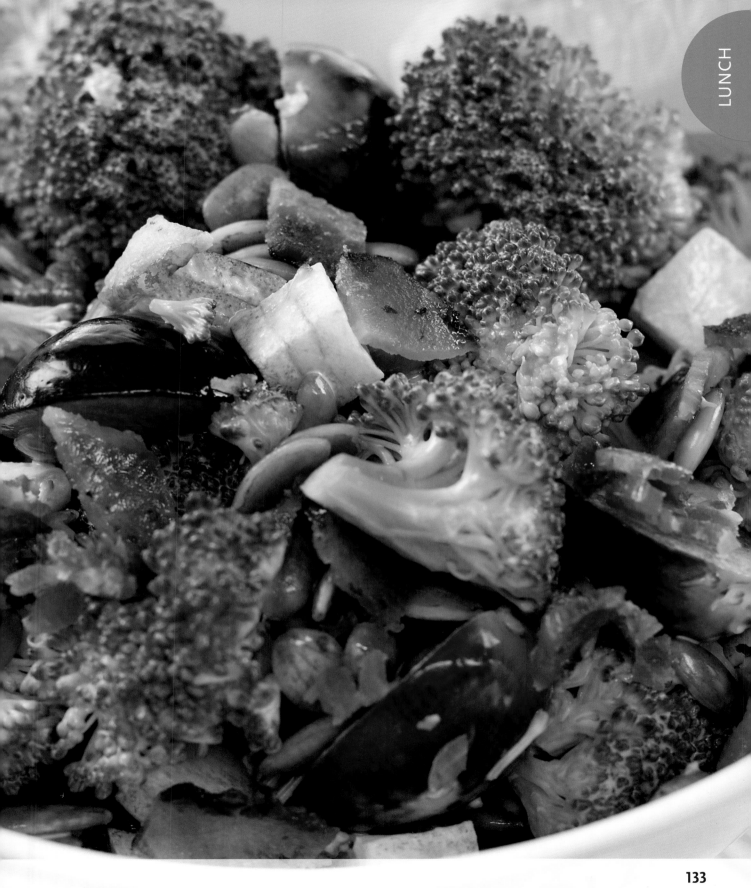

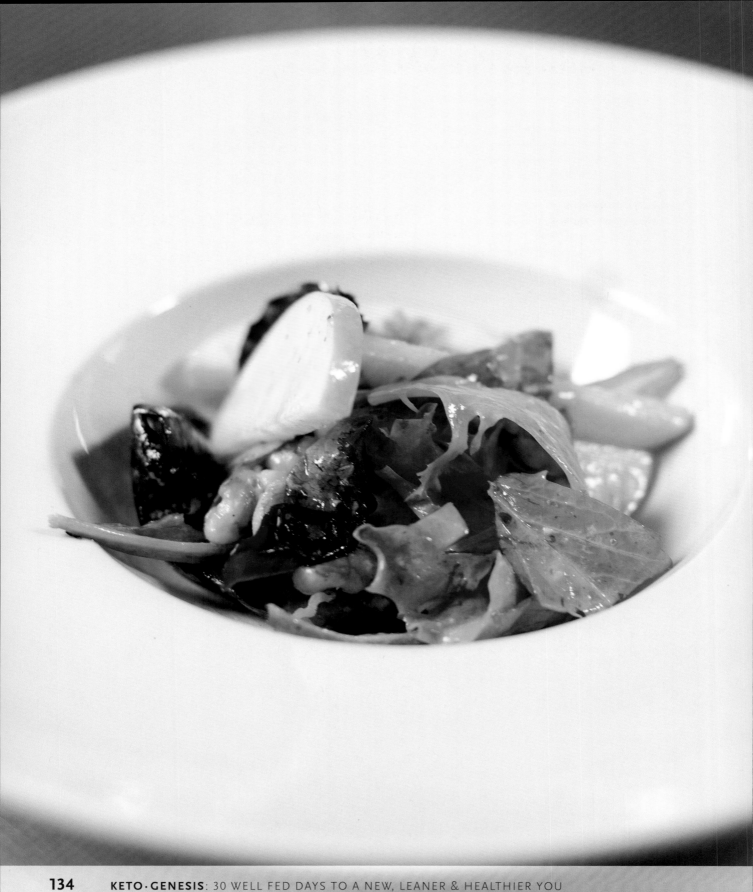

WALNUT AND APPLE SALAD with Blue Cheese Dressing

Serves 2 | Ready in 15 minutes

SALAD

400g mixed greens
200g walnuts, toasted
100g green apples, chopped

DRESSING

50g blue cheese
45 mL Alpha Balance™ Oil or olive oil
30 mL fresh lemon juice
5g fresh dill
3g fresh thyme
5 mL Dijon mustard
5 mL Tabasco sauce
Salt and pepper

Delicious with barbequed steak. —AT

IN a pan on low heat, gently toast the walnuts until aromatic, and then let cool.

BLEND all of the dressing ingredients in a blender until smooth.

TOSS the mixed greens, apples and walnuts with dressing in a large bowl.

SEASON with salt and pepper, and serve.

NET CARBS 15.3G	PROTEIN 23.8G PER SERVING

GF   VEG

WALNUT HUMMUS CUCUMBER CANOES

Serves 2 | Ready in 15 minutes

200g raw walnuts

120 mL olive oil

12g (4 small cloves) garlic

25g nutritional yeast

30 mL fresh lemon juice

50g fresh basil

1 pinch of red pepper flakes

Salt and pepper to taste

4 small cucumbers, halved and seeded
  (like little canoes)

PULSE all ingredients except cucumbers in a food processor, until the consistency of hummus is reached.

FILL cucumbers with walnut hummus and serve.

NET CARBS 15.2G	PROTEIN 21.8G PER SERVING

 GF   VEGAN   DAIRY FREE   VEG

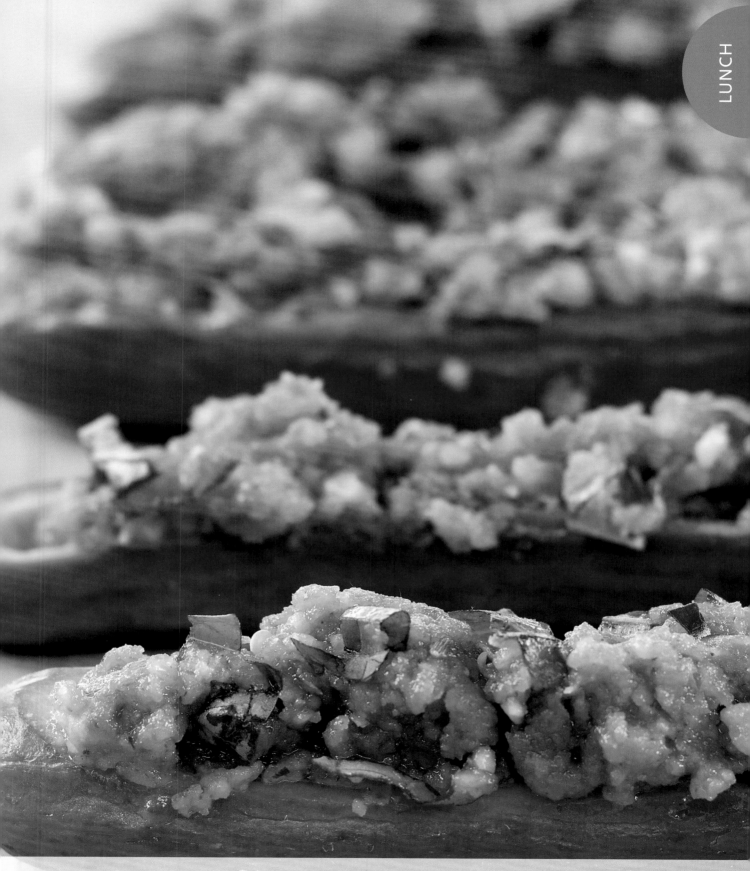

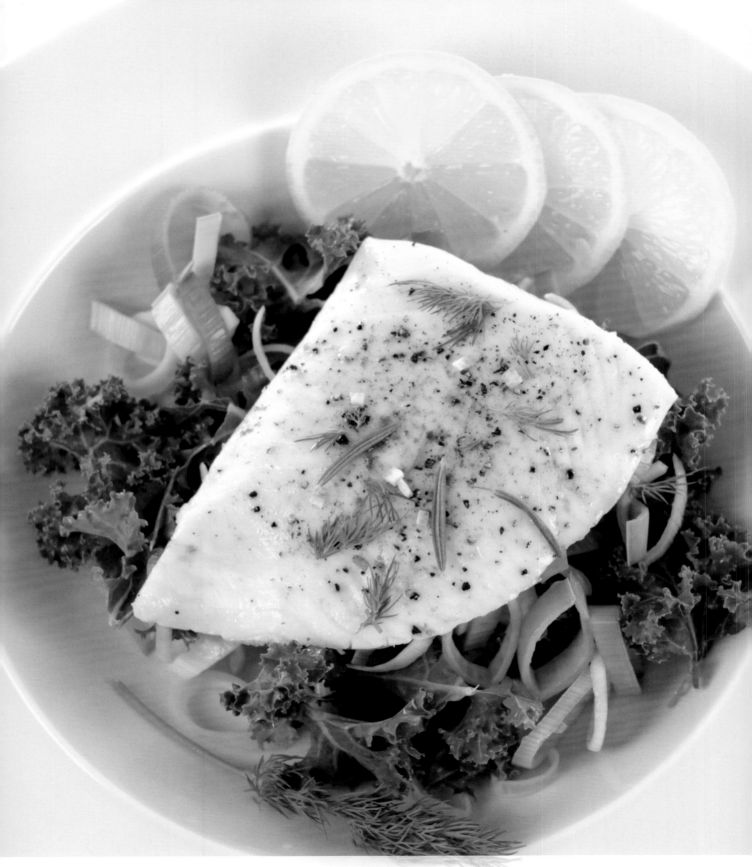

WARM LEEK AND KALE SALAD with Baked Halibut Steaks

Serves 4 | Ready in 35 minutes

SALAD

15g butter
10g (3 small cloves) garlic, sliced
200g leeks, washed and chopped
2g fresh thyme, chopped
1.5 mL sweet paprika
350g green kale, washed, spines removed,
    and roughly chopped
1 lemon, juiced
Salt and pepper to taste

HALIBUT STEAKS

2 lemons
1.5g of fresh dill
30 mL butter, melted
900g (4 steaks) halibut
4 rosemary sprigs
Sea salt and ground pepper to taste

SALAD

IN a large sauce pan, heat butter on medium heat.

ADD garlic and cook until fragrant. Add the leeks, thyme, and paprika, sauté for 10 minutes until soft. Add kale and lemon juice, and cook for 5 minutes longer.

REMOVE from heat, plate, and top with halibut steaks.

PREHEAT oven to 230°C (450°F).

HALIBUT STEAKS

USING a lemon zester, or the smallest hole on your cheese grater, zest both lemons.

COMBINE lemon zest, the juice from lemons, dill, and butter in a small bowl and whisk.

RUB butter mixture into steaks and marinate for twenty minutes.

PLACE rosemary along base of a shallow baking dish and place halibut steaks on top. Pour any leftover butter mixture over the halibut.

BAKE for 15–20 minutes and serve with salad.

NET CARBS 17G	PROTEIN 51G PER SERVING

GF

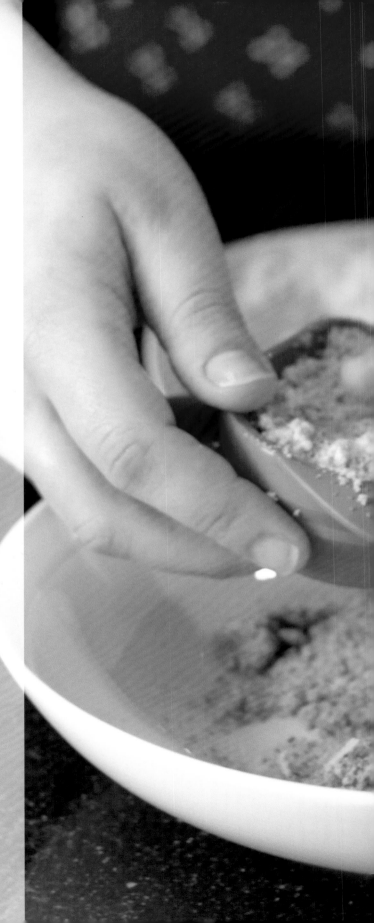

DINNER & DESSERTS

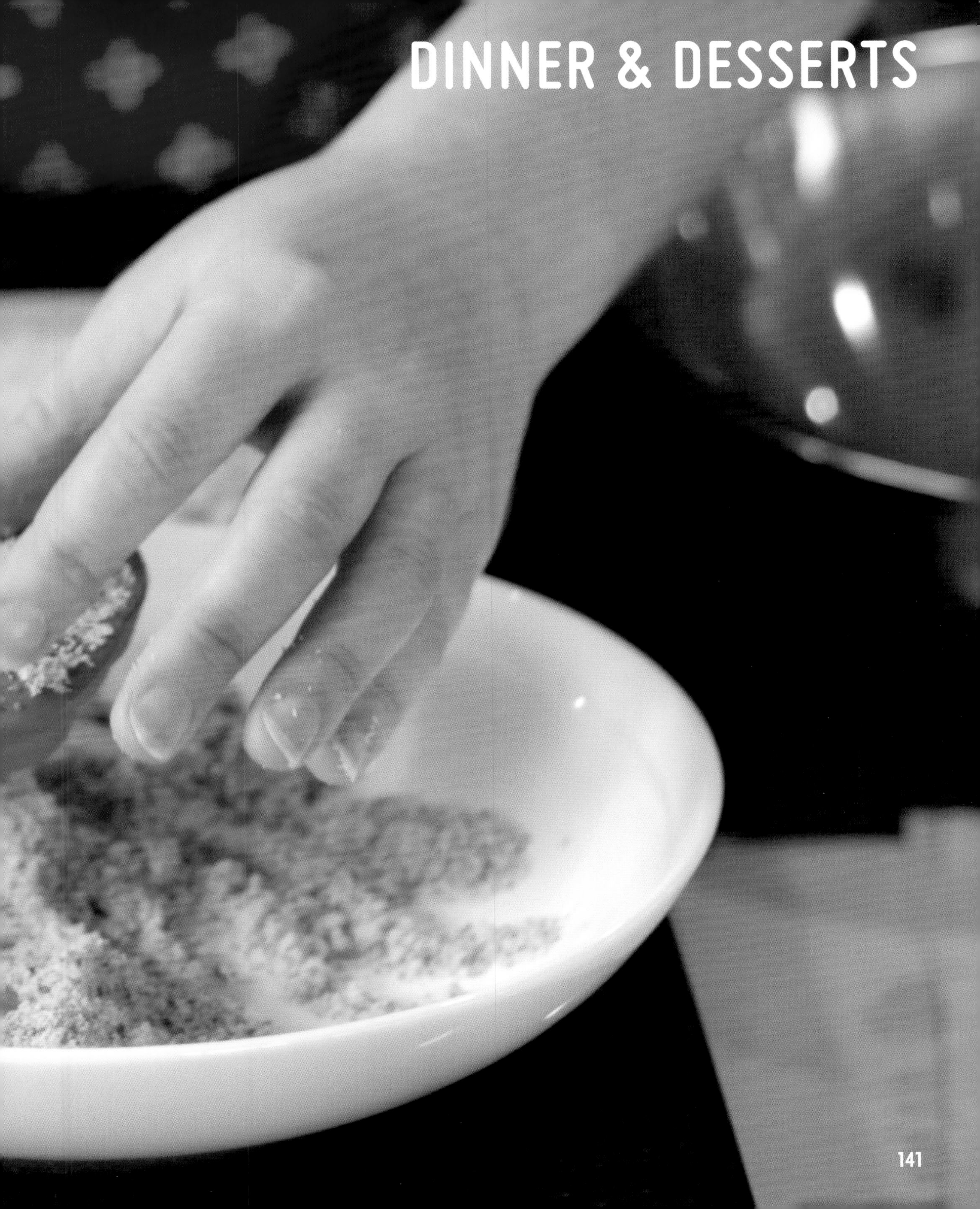

ASIAN LETTUCE WRAPS

Serves 4 | Ready in 25 minutes

25g pecans

15 mL red palm olein

9g (3 cloves) garlic, minced

250g (2 breasts) chicken, cut into bite-size
    pieces

15g ginger, thinly sliced

50g onion, chopped

250g water chestnuts, sliced into
    matchsticks

200g shiitake mushrooms, sliced into
    matchsticks

30 mL Bragg's soy seasoning

30 mL peanut butter

5 mL crushed chili flakes

10 mL rice vinegar

5 mL Thai Curry Paste (page 218)

8g coconut sugar

50g red bell pepper, chopped

2g green onions, thinly sliced

6–10 whole lettuce leaves for wrapping

TOAST pecans lightly either in a skillet or toaster oven.

IN a skillet, heat palm olein, add sliced ginger and saute until fragrant. Add minced garlic and saute until fragrant. Add chicken and stir-fry until cooked through.

ADD onion, chestnut, and mushroom. Sauté for 2 minutes.

IN a separate bowl, combine Bragg's, peanut butter, chili flakes, vinegar, curry paste, and coconut sugar. Add red pepper to pan, then pour mixture over chicken and cook for 2 more minutes.

REMOVE from heat and stir in the green onions.

ASSEMBLE by placing chicken stir fry into lettuce leaf and top with pecans.

NET CARBS 14G	PROTEIN 16.4G PER SERVING

 GF   DAIRY FREE

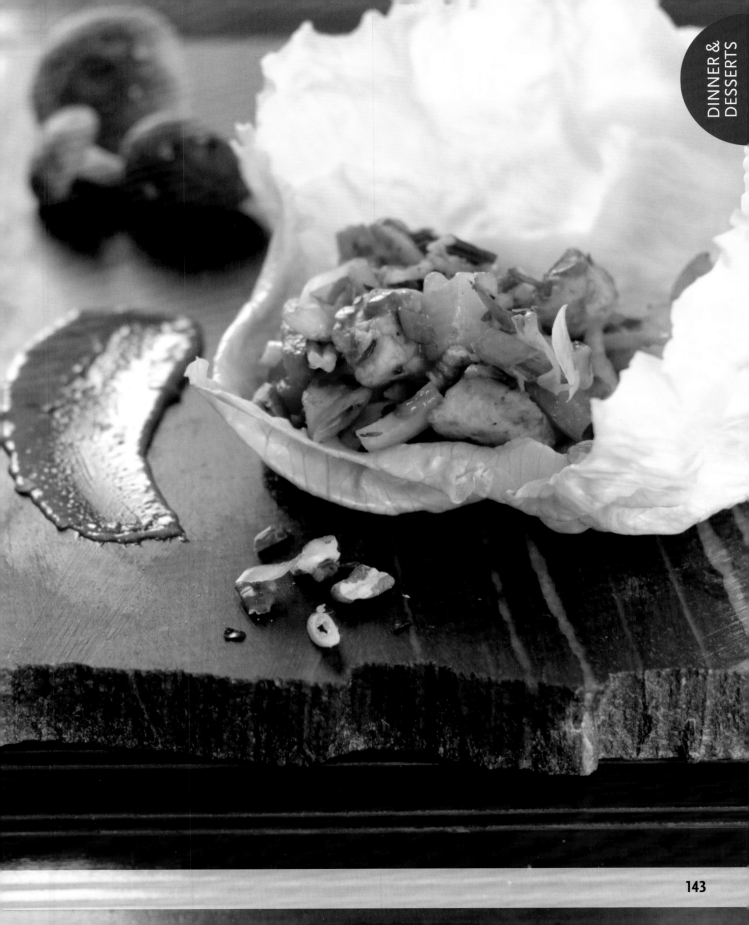

DINNER &
DESSERTS

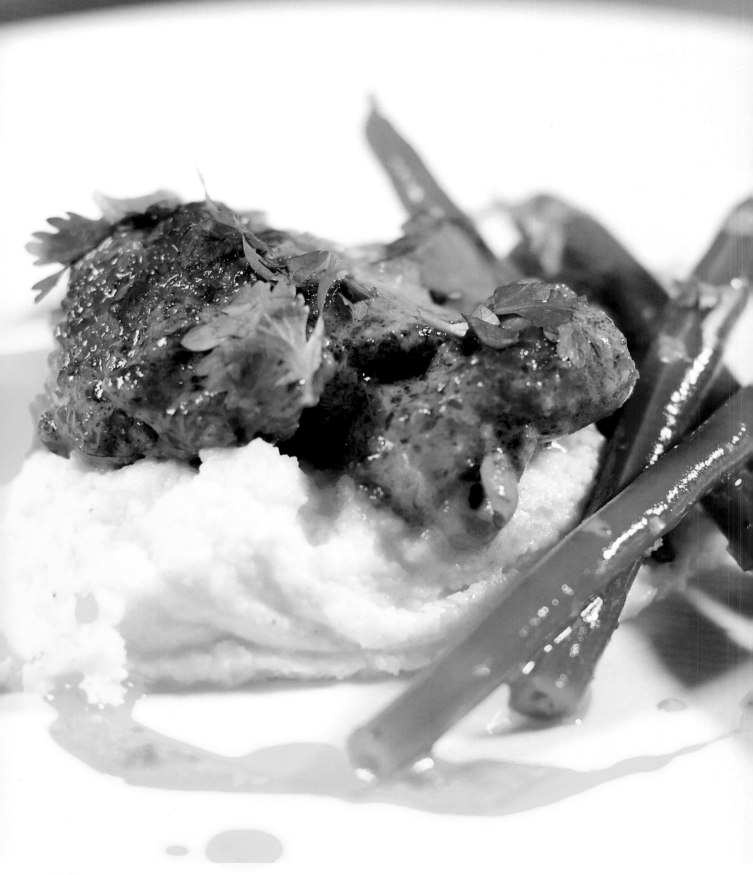

BRAISED BASIL MINT CHICKEN

Serves 4 | Ready in 1.5 hours

15g fresh basil

8g fresh mint

30g fresh ginger

18g (6 cloves) garlic

1 Thai chili

5 mL coarse salt

60 mL Alpha Balance™ Oil

5 mL DME™ Coconut Oil

8 chicken thighs, bone-in

250 mL chicken stock

125 mL amber rum

60 mL heavy (whipping) cream

30 mL lemon juice

This recipe is adapted from Molly Stevens, and has become a family favourite. We usually have fresh basil around the house, but not so with fresh mint. So I'll substitute a teabag of peppermint tea. Thanks, James Barber. −CG

COMBINE basil, mint, ginger, garlic, chili, salt and Alpha Balance™ Oil in blender, and blend into a smooth paste. Put into freezer storage bag with chicken thighs, and massage to thoroughly coat chicken. Marinate for 30 minutes.

HEAT the coconut oil in a large pan (a dutch oven works well – it must have a tight fitting lid) until it shimmers. Place the chicken skin side down and brown, then turn and brown other side. Remove from pan and set aside on plate to catch drippings. Pour off the excess oil from the pan.

DEGLAZE the pan with rum, and reduce to half. Scrape out remaining marinade and add it to the pan. Add chicken stock, and bring to a boil. Turn down to low (simmer if your range has that option), add chicken with drippings, cover tightly. Turn chicken after 15 minutes. Simmer for another 15 minutes until done, or until inserted thermometer reads 75°C (170°F).

REMOVE the chicken and set aside under foil. Bring liquid to boil to reduce, then add heavy cream. Add 30 mL lemon juice to brighten sauce. Serve sauce over chicken.

 When planning your cooking time, be sure to account for two 30-minute interludes in this recipe – the marinating and the braising. This is a meal that freezes well, if you have to cook ahead.

NET CARBS 4.3G	PROTEIN 27.9G PER SERVING

GF

BRAISED CARIBBEAN CHICKEN

Serves 6 | Ready in 65 minutes

10 allspice berries

16 peppercorns

4 cloves (whole)

1 chicken, separated (or parts, bone in, skin on)

30 mL DME™ Coconut Oil or red palm olein

225g celery, chopped

200g bell pepper, chopped coarse

2.5 mL cumin

2.5 mL pepper flakes

2.5 mL cardamom

2.5 mL cinnamon

275g onion, chopped coarse

250 mL chicken or vegetable stock

125 mL rum

5 mL salt

GRIND the allspice, peppercorns, and cloves in a spice grinder or with mortar and pestle.

DRY off chicken pieces with paper towel. Heat the coconut oil in a 30cm skillet (must have a tight fitting lid) over medium until oil shimmers. Place the chicken pieces skin side down, turning when browned, about 5 minutes per side. Set the chicken aside on a plate to catch the drippings.

ADD the onions, celery, and peppers to the hot pan. Add the spices and salt, and sauté until the onions are soft. Deglaze the pan with the rum. Add the stock and bring to a boil to meld flavours. Turn down to simmer. Add the chicken pieces skin side down and cover with the lid. Simmer for 20 minutes, turn the chicken skin side up, and simmer for another 20 minutes until done, or until an inserted thermometer reads 75°C (170°F).

REMOVE the chicken pieces and cover with foil to keep warm. Bring the sauce to a boil, and reduce to your desired consistency. Place vegetable sauce on warmed dish, top with chicken, and serve.

 Caribbean dishes are typically made with onions, celery, and green bell peppers, but I prefer the red, both for colour and for flavour.

NET CARBS 6.1G   PROTEIN 19.3G PER SERVING

 GF   DAIRY FREE

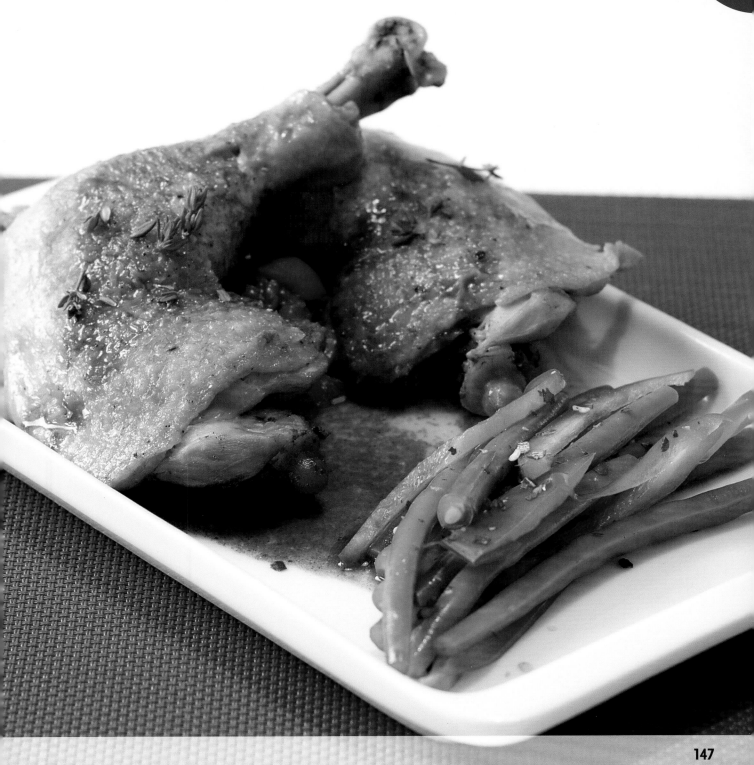

BEEF TENDERLOIN with Horseradish Cauliflower Mash

Serves 2 | Ready in 45 minutes

30 mL butter, reserve half for cauliflower

6g (2 small cloves) garlic, minced

15 mL balsamic vinegar

5 mL Dijon mustard

5 mL kosher salt

230g (2 steaks) beef tenderloin

500g cauliflower, chopped and steamed

30 mL cream

15 mL prepared horseradish

25g flat leaf parsley, chopped

Salt and pepper to taste

This is a new take on a childhood favourite, roast beef with horseradish. — AT

PREHEAT oven to 220°C (425°F).

IN a small dish combine 15 mL butter, garlic, balsamic vinegar, and Dijon mustard until a thick paste. Rub both sides of each steak with the mixture and then sprinkle with kosher salt. Set aside.

IN a large pot, steam and drain cauliflower. Add cauliflower back to warm pot and on low heat, add remaining butter, horseradish, and cream. Purée with an immersion blender until creamy. Do not over purée; it should be the consistency of mashed potatoes. Fold in fresh parsley and season to taste.

IN a cast iron skillet on medium high heat, sear steaks on both sides.

REMOVE skillet from stove top and place in pre-heated oven. For medium rare meat, cook for 7 minutes, and cook for 10 minutes for medium well meat. Let tenderloin rest for 5 minutes before serving.

PLATE cauliflower mash and top with steaks. Season with fresh ground pepper and a sprinkle of salt.

 You can prepare your own horseradish. The fresher it is, the more potent it will be. Use 3.75 mL vinegar for every 25 mL of grated horseradish. Wait at least 3 minutes after grating for "heat" to develop. The longer you wait, the more the heat diminishes. For a softer flavour, you can prepare horseradish in heavy cream.

NET CARBS 10.8G   PROTEIN 35G PER SERVING

GF

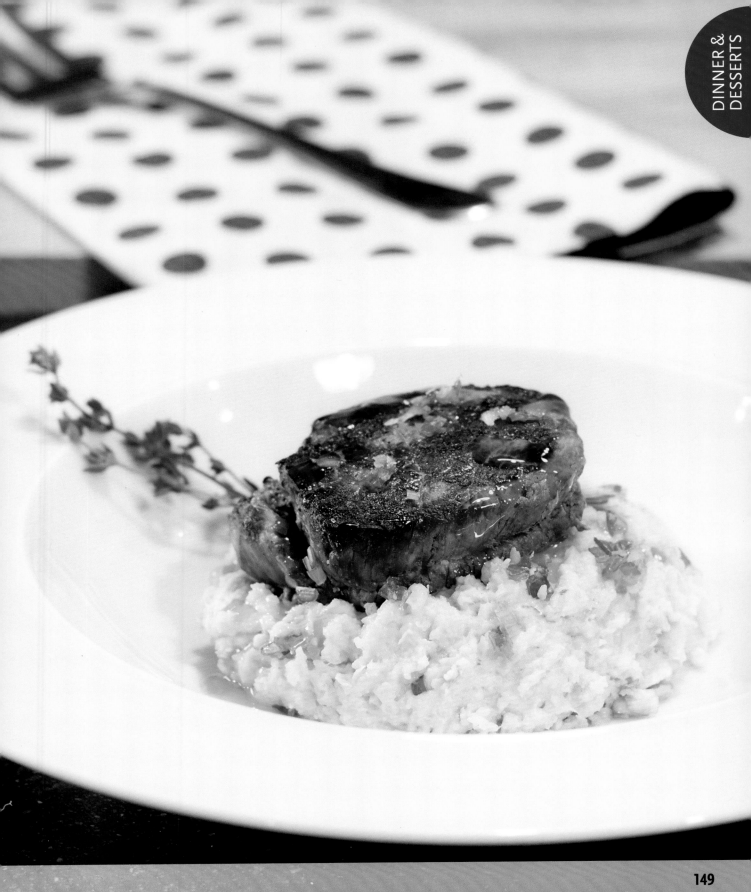

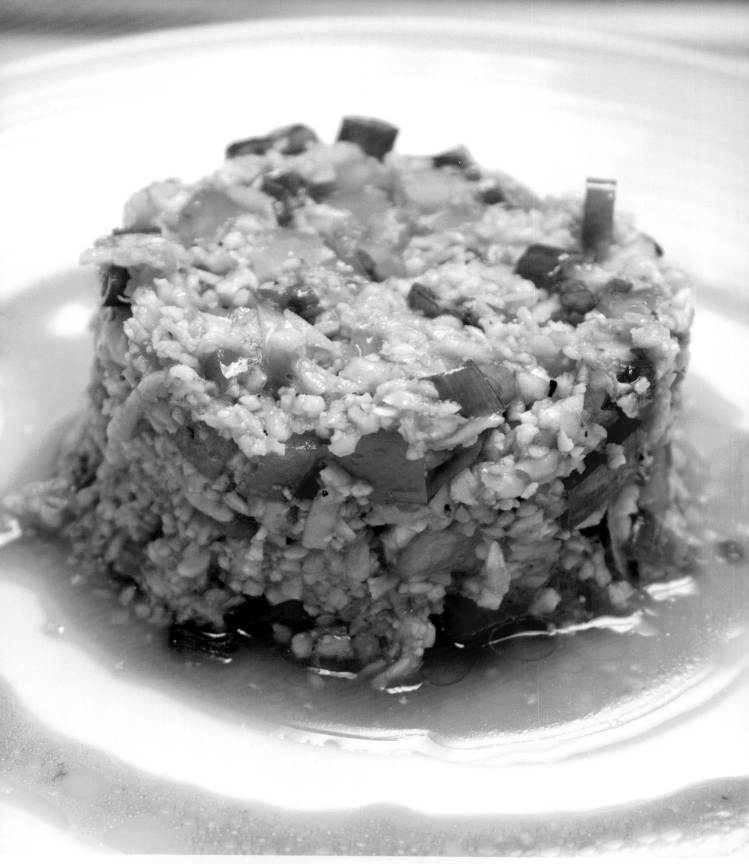

CAULIFLOWER COUSCOUS SALAD with Hazelnut Coconut Cod

Serves 4 | Ready in 45 minutes

VINAIGRETTE

175 mL Alpha Balance™ Oil
Zest and juice of 2 limes
6g (2 small cloves) garlic, minced
2g coconut sugar
30 mL balsamic vinegar
Salt and pepper to taste

SALAD

400g cauliflower florets, grated
200g assorted bell peppers, diced
250g tomato, diced
75g green onions, thinly sliced
30g slivered almonds, toasted

COD

500g (4 filets) cod
60g hazelnuts, ground
20g coconut flour
8g parsley, chopped
2g thyme, chopped
2.5 mL salt
Pinch of black pepper, ground
1 lemon, zested
120 mL coconut milk for wash

This is a recipe Chef Tom Liu created for Alpha Health Products using Alpha Balance™ Oil. We liked the idea of gluten-free couscous so much, we adapted it for our cookbook. —CG

VINAIGRETTE

COMBINE all ingredients for vinaigrette and whisk thoroughly.

SALAD

COMBINE all couscous salad ingredients and mix with vinaigrette. Allow to sit for 20 minutes to infuse flavours.

COD

PREHEAT oven to 205°C (400°F).

DRY filet. Cut into portion sizes.

COMBINE hazelnuts, coconut flour, herbs, salt, pepper, and lemon zest.

DIP filet in coconut milk, then dredge in hazelnut mixture. Place on baking pan.

BAKE for 15 minutes. Finish with a squeeze of lemon juice.

NET CARBS 14.5G	PROTEIN 29.5G PER SERVING

 GF DAIRY FREE

CAULIFLOWER CRUST PIZZA

Serves 4 | Ready in 50 minutes

275g (1 small head) cauliflower
1 egg
170g Mozzarella cheese, grated
5 mL oregano, ground
100g onion, minced
3g (1 clove) garlic, minced
5 mL salt

125 mL Barbeque Sauce (page 215)
100g grape tomatoes, halved
200g grilled chicken, chopped
150g Mozzarella, grated

PREHEAT oven to 205°C (400°F).

CRUST

STEAM cauliflower with a minimal amount of water. Cauliflower should be fairly dry when done. Purée cauliflower in food processor.

COMBINE cauliflower, egg, Mozzarella, oregano, onion, garlic, and salt in a medium mixing bowl.

TRANSFER to parchment-lined baking sheet and smooth out to ½ inch or thinner.

BAKE for 20–25 minutes until slightly golden.

PIZZA

REMOVE the crust from the oven. Top the crust with Barbeque Sauce (page 215), toppings and cheese.

PLACE back in the oven for 20 minutes or until cheese is melted.

 You can make four mini pizza crusts rather than one large crust. After baking and cooling, wrap individually and freeze for a day you want a quick pizza!

NET CARBS 9.1G   PROTEIN 37G PER SERVING

GF

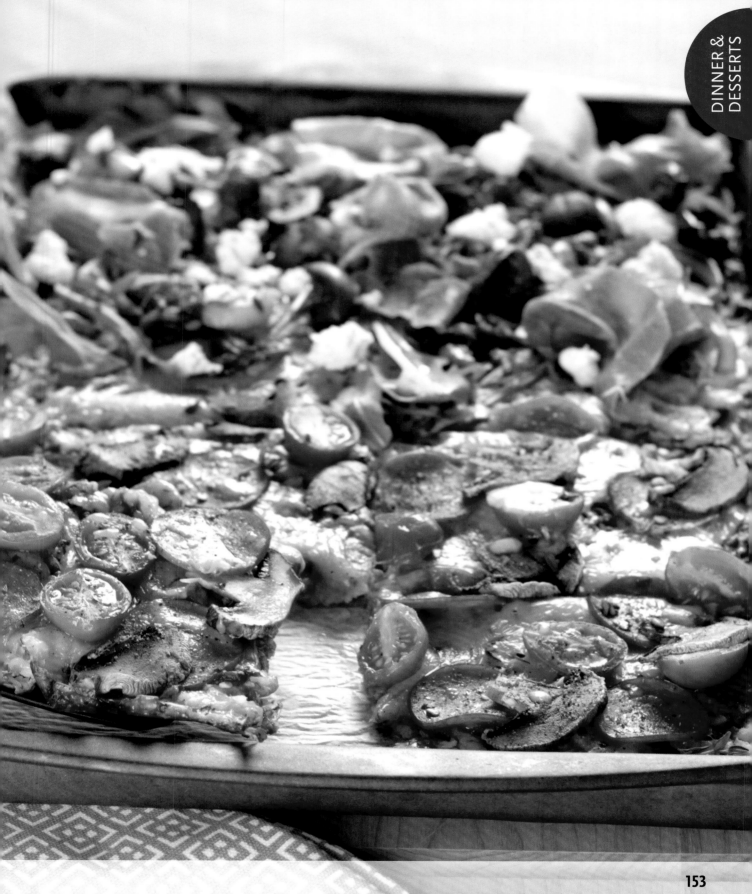

CHRISTEL'S NUT FALAFEL

Serves 4 | Ready in 40 minutes

200g carrots
100g almonds
150g hazelnuts
150g onion
6g (2 cloves) garlic, minced
30 mL Bragg's soy seasoning
45 mL tomato paste
30 mL Alpha Balance™ Oil or camelina oil
15g fresh parsley
5g fresh thyme
5g fresh oregano
2.5 mL coriander
2.5 mL ground mustard
2.5 mL salt
1.25 mL white pepper
125 mL DME™ Coconut Oil for frying
(enough to cover the pan ½ cm deep)

Originally a recipe to use up the remains of juicing carrots, it has morphed into this great vegan taste sensation. Then again, a lot of recipes that taste fabulous started out with "how do I make use of this…" – CG

PREHEAT oven to 190°C (375°F).

GRATE the carrots fine or use a food processor to get them really fine.

GRIND the nuts in a blender or food processor.

CHOP the onions fine and sauté until soft. Add the minced garlic and sauté until fragrant.

COMBINE with the grated carrots, ground nuts, oil and chopped herbs and spices. Mix with a spatula until thoroughly blended.

FORM the mixture into balls and set aside on parchment paper.

HEAT the oil in a heavy pan over scant medium heat, until the oil shimmers. Turn down the heat slightly and let pan gather heat for five minutes. Turn the heat back to medium and brown the falafel balls on three sides. Set on a baking sheet.

BAKE for 15 minutes, until heated through.

NET CARBS 12G	PROTEIN 21.6G PER SERVING

 GF   VEGAN   DAIRY FREE VEG

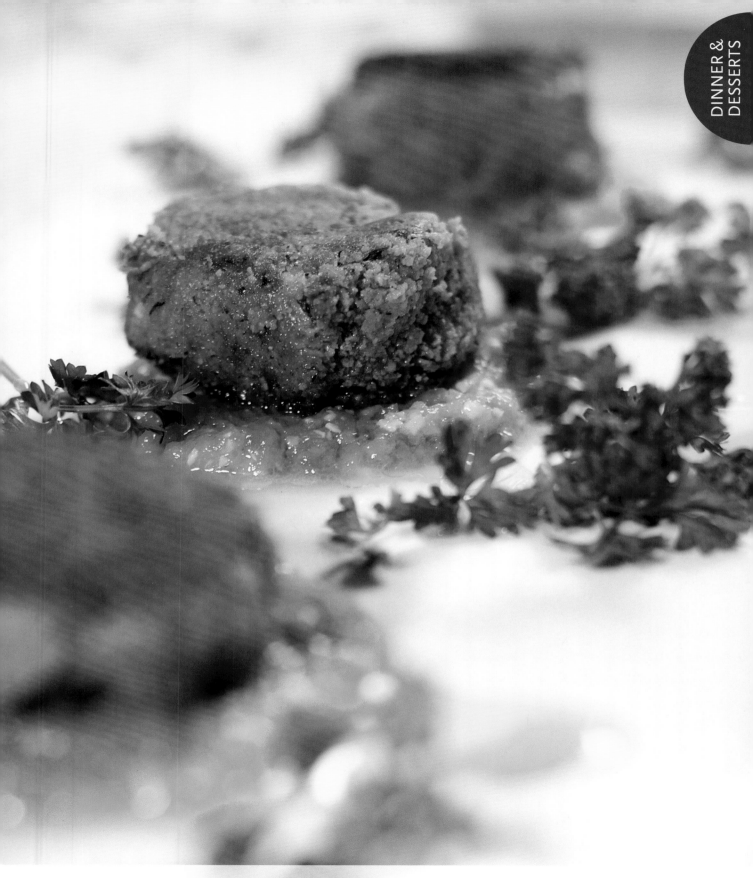

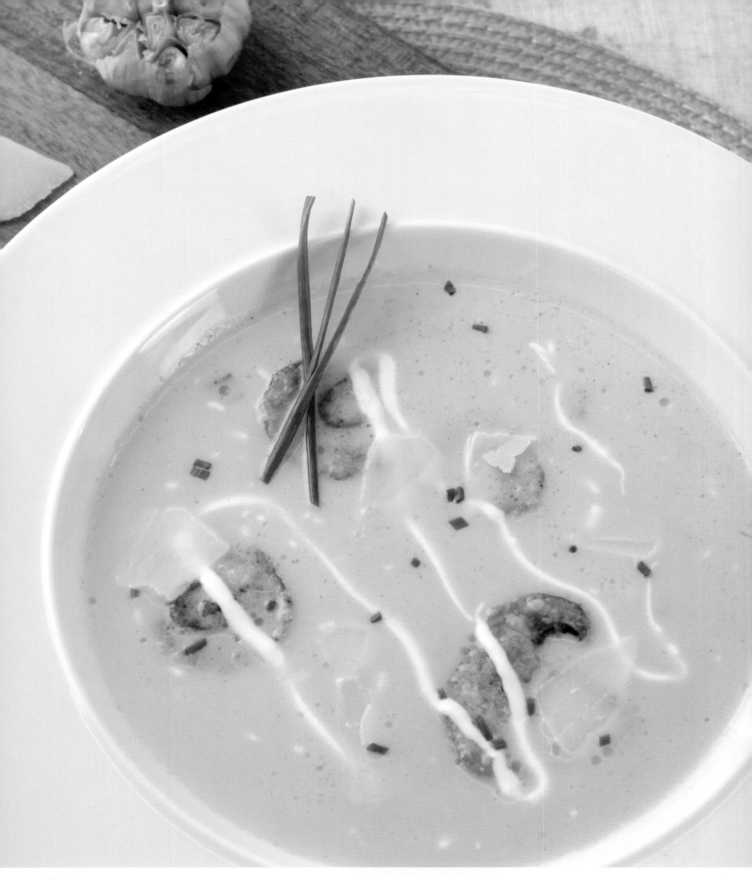

CREAMY ROAST GARLIC SOUP with Parmesan Mushrooms

Serves 4 | Ready in 45 minutes

4 garlic bulbs, tops chopped off so cloves
  are exposed

30 mL camelina oil

15 mL butter

50g sweet onion, diced

100g celery, diced

100g carrots, diced

1 bay leaf

10 mL sweet smoked paprika

1L vegetable stock, chicken stock or
  beef stock

5g arrowroot starch

30 mL cold water

80 mL cream

30 mL fresh chives, chopped

60 mL thick Greek (10% mf) yogurt

80g white or brown mushrooms, halved

50g of Parmesan cheese, grated

1.25 mL oregano

Salt and pepper to taste

PREHEAT oven to 175°C (350°F). In a small baking dish, drizzle garlic bulbs in camelina oil, and roast 30 minutes or until soft.

REMOVE garlic from oven and let cool.

IN a heavy sauce pan, melt butter over medium heat. Add onions, celery, carrots, and garlic. Sauté until soft.

ADD bay leaf, paprika, and vegetable stock.

DISSOLVE arrowroot powder in cold water and add to pot. Bring to a boil, stirring often, and reduce heat to low. Add cream and purée with an immersion blender. Keep warm, stirring often.

TURN on broiler.

IN a small bowl, toss mushrooms in a bit of butter or camelina oil, cheese, oregano, and salt and pepper. Spread out on a baking sheet.

POP mushrooms under broiler for 2 minutes until brown.

TOP bowls of soup with fresh chives, a dollop of Greek yogurt, and the Parmesan Mushrooms.

NET CARBS 15.4G	PROTEIN 10.4G PER SERVING

 GF   VEG

CREOLE PRAWNS WITH YAM LATKES

Serves 4 | Ready in 35 minutes

LATKES

150g yam, peeled & grated
20g onion, diced
25g coconut flour
1 egg
5 mL salt
30 mL milk
15 mL DME™ Coconut Oil

PRAWNS

30 mL DME™ Coconut Oil
40g onion, diced
15g (5 cloves) garlic, sliced
5g oregano, chopped
5g thyme, chopped
15 mL cracked black pepper
5 mL coarse sea salt
2.5 mL cayenne pepper or to taste
350g (32 medium) prawns, peeled &
    deveined, thawed
50g scallions, chopped
Dash of cognac
50g parsley, chopped

Lemon and lime wedges for serving

LATKES

COMBINE the grated yam, onion, coconut flour, egg, and salt in a bowl. Add just enough milk to moisten the mixture to the point where patties hold together.

HEAT the coconut oil in a cast iron frying pan over medium high heat. When the oil begins to shimmer, lay the patties in the pan. Fry approximately 3 minutes, until the edges begin to brown. Flip gently, and fry for another 3 minutes, until done. Remove from heat and cover until served.

PRAWNS

HEAT the coconut oil in a frying pan over medium heat. When the oil begins to shimmer, add the onions and fry gently until soft (about 3 minutes). Turn the heat down to medium low and add the garlic.

MIX the oregano, thyme, black pepper, cayenne, and salt in a bowl large enough to hold all the prawns. Add the prawns and toss to coat. Place the prawns in the frying pan. When the underside becomes translucent, turn.

WHEN prawns are cooked, pink and firm, add a dash of cognac to the pan to deglaze. The alcohol will reduce very quickly. When about half the amount remains, empty the contents of the pan into your serving dish.

ADD the chopped scallions (green onions). You may toss if you wish. Cover the dish with chopped parsley. Drizzle the lemon/lime juice on top, and garnish with wedges.

 Serve with sour cream or tzatziki.

NET CARBS 15.3G	PROTEIN 20.7G PER SERVING

 GF   DAIRY FREE

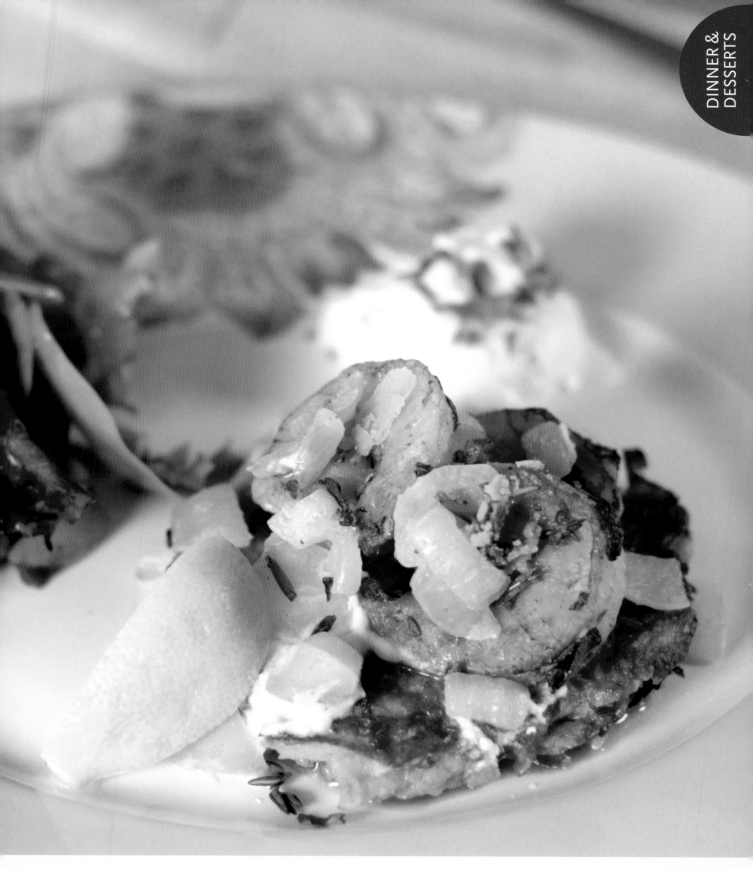

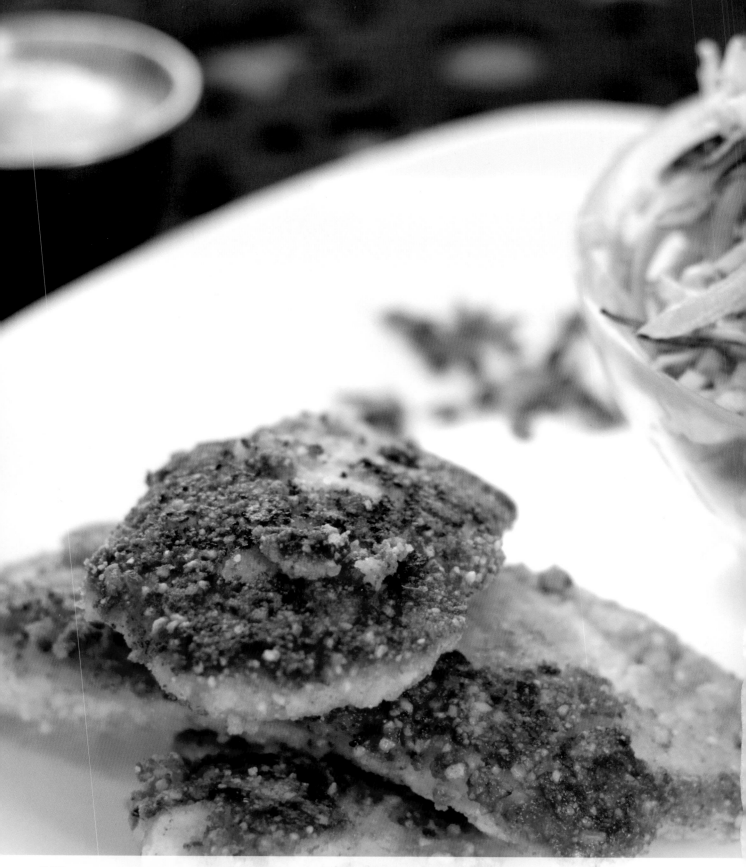

CRISPY FRIED CHICKEN with Creamy Coleslaw

Serves 4 | Ready in 45 minutes

DINNER & DESSERTS

- 500g (4 medium) boneless, skinless chicken breasts
- 250 mL buttermilk
- 15 mL Dijon mustard
- 75g almond flour
- 30g coconut flour
- 15 mL ground pepper
- 5 mL salt
- 2.5 mL cayenne pepper
- 5 mL dried oregano
- 5 mL dried thyme
- 5 mL garlic powder
- 5 mL onion powder

- 250 mL DME™ Coconut Oil or red palm oil, for frying

This meal was one of my favourite to create, and eat. You could use the fried chicken in a lettuce wrap or topped on a fresh salad. —AT

RINSE chicken, pat dry, and slice into evenly sized strips.

MIX buttermilk and Dijon mustard together in a small bowl. Season with a pinch of salt and pepper.

PLACE chicken in a large plastic bag and cover with buttermilk mixture.

MARINATE for 15–45 minutes.

IN a clean bowl, add remaining ingredients and stir.

REMOVE chicken from marinade and coat each piece in the flour mixture.

HEAT oil on medium high heat and fry chicken until evenly browned on both sides. Remove and drain on a paper towel.

PLATE with coleslaw (see below).

 You can skip the buttermilk soak and just dip chicken in an egg bath before coating.

NET CARBS 7.8G	PROTEIN 29G PER SERVING

 GF

CREAMY COLESLAW

Serves 4 | Ready in 20 minutes

- 400g green and red cabbage, shredded
- 100g carrots, shredded
- 250 mL Greek (10% mf) yogurt
- 50g Spanish/sweet onion, diced
- 15 mL unrefined apple cider vinegar
- 15 mL Dijon mustard
- 5 mL celery salt
- 5 mL honey
- Salt and pepper to taste (just before serving)

IN a small bowl, whisk yogurt, mustard, vinegar, and honey. Toss vegetables with dressing, and season to taste. Refrigerate until ready to serve. Generously season with fresh ground pepper and sea salt.

NET CARBS 8.9G	PROTEIN 7.6G PER SERVING

 GF   VEG

161

DAIKON HASH

Serves 4 | Ready in 30 minutes

100g mushrooms, sliced
45 mL red palm olein
400g daikon, cubed ½ cm
175g Napa cabbage, shredded
100g celery, sliced thin
40g green onions, sliced
2 bay leaves
125 mL hard apple cider
60 mL vegetable stock
2.5 mL black pepper, fresh coarse ground
3.5 mL salt

One of the challenges of switching over to a ketogenic way of eating is replacing the starch dishes we're so fond of in our culture. Daikon hash is a great accompaniment to your protein of choice. – CG

SAUTÉ the mushrooms over medium high heat in 30 mL palm olein in a 25 cm skillet. Add 1 mL of the salt and all of the pepper. When mushrooms have browned, remove from heat and set aside in a bowl.

ADD remaining palm olein to pan. Add daikon and brown. Add cabbage, celery, and bay leaves, and sauté for 10 minutes. Add the stock, cider, and salt, stir briefly and cover. Turn down heat and let cook until daikon can be pierced with a fork. Cook briefly without a lid to cook off remaining liquid.

TURN off heat, remove the bay leaves, add the mushrooms and the green onions, toss, and serve.

TIP This hash can be made with butter instead of red palm olein for a richer dish.

NET CARBS 9.2G	PROTEIN 2.7G PER SERVING

 GF   VEGAN   DAIRY FREE   VEG

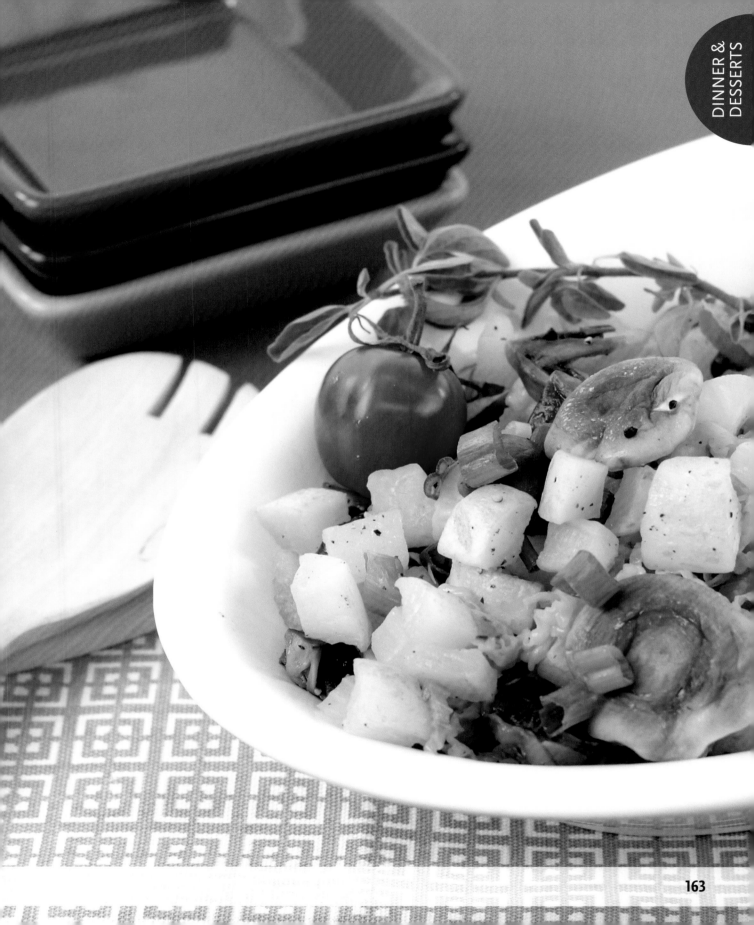

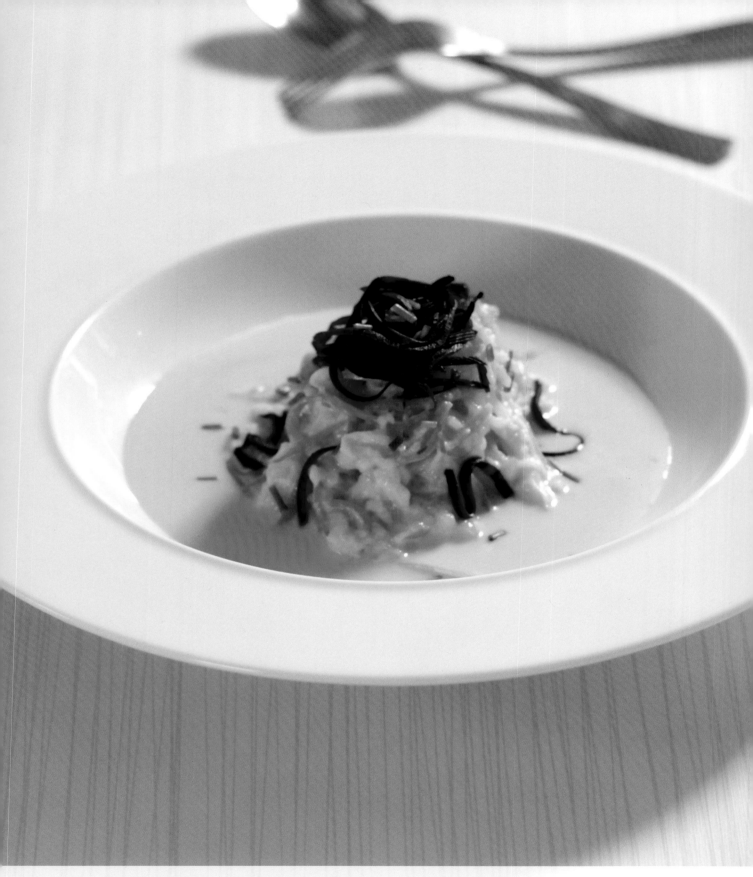

FIVE CHEESE VEGGETINI ALFREDO

Serves 4 | Ready in 25 minutes

200g daikon, julienned

200g carrot, julienned

100g beet, julienned (optional)

250 mL heavy cream (reduced) or
    125 mL heavy cream

150g cheese (Parmesan, aged Cheddar,
    Gruyère, Ementhal, or Gouda)

1 egg

15 mL Alpha Balance™ Oil

2.5 mL salt

1.25 mL black pepper, fresh ground

Dash of nutmeg

REDUCE 250 mL of heavy cream to half for a richer flavour. If you are short on time, bring 125 mL of cream to a quick boil.

GRATE cheese with fine grater. Optionally set aside some cheese to sprinkle on top. Mix egg thoroughly into the rest of grated cheese.

LIGHTLY sauté julienned vegetables in oil for 3 minutes. Vegetables should be warmed through but still al dente. Turn off heat. Add cream to pan. Add salt, pepper and nutmeg. Toss. Add cheese mixture and stir to combine until cheese is thoroughly melted. The heat of the cream will cook the egg. Note: if you do add beets, the entire dish will have a pink hue.

SPRINKLE reserved cheese on top and serve.

 Reducing the cream adds complexity to the flavour, and thickness to the sauce. Although you can make the dish without it, and it's still tasty, the step is highly recommended.

NET CARBS 13.2G	PROTEIN 15G PER SERVING

GF   VEG

HORSERADISH CREAM OF BEET SOUP

Serves 4 | Ready in 35 minutes

10g horseradish, finely grated
250 mL half & half cream
200g beets, peeled and cubed to 1 cm
250 mL vegetable broth
Boiled water to taste
½ lemon, zested
Salt to taste

I know I've come up with a good recipe when I can't stop eating until the bowl is empty. The beets, the lemon, the horseradish — it all comes together. This may not be the soup to make if you want a lot of conversation. —CG

MIX horseradish with a splash of the cream, and set aside.

BOIL beets with vegetable broth in tightly covered pot until soft, about 25 minutes.

PURÉE in blender, or with immersion blender.

RETURN to pot on simmer, and add boiling water to bring total to 500 mL.

ADD horseradish mixture to cream and stir into soup. The soup should have the consistency to coat the back of a spoon.

ADD lemon zest and salt to taste.

NET CARBS 5.9G	PROTEIN 2.3G PER SERVING

 GF   VEG

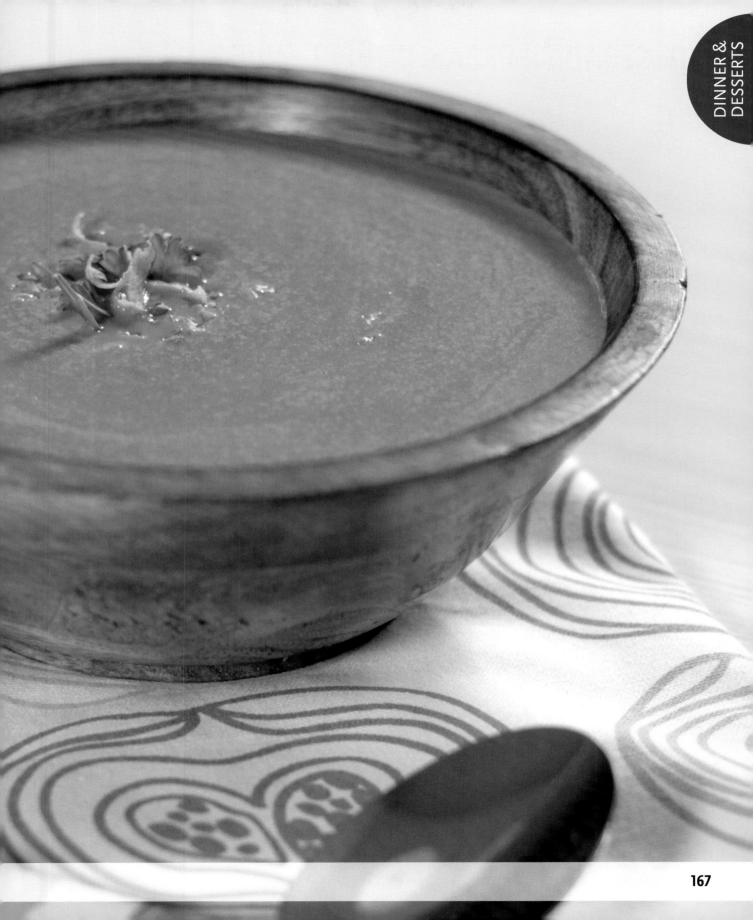

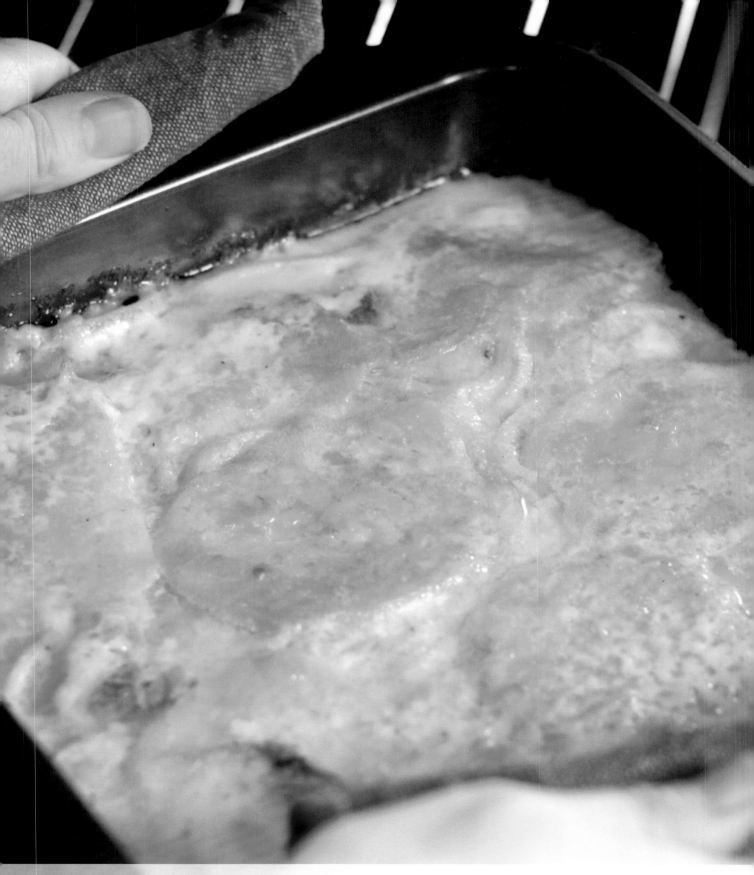

KOHLRABI GRATIN

Serves 4 | Ready in 1 hour 15 minutes

30g Parmesan cheese

30g Gouda cheese

30g aged Cheddar

15g butter

100g onion, peeled, sliced thin

400g kohlrabi, peeled, sliced thin

5 mL salt

5 mL pepper

15g flour

250 mL heavy (whipping) cream

There are plenty of low carbohydrate vegetables. We just need to find flavourful ways of preparing them. The kohlrabi retains just a bit of firmness, giving this dish the right texture and mouth feel. — CG

GRATE cheese fine. Grease bottom of 8" square baking dish with butter. Lay out ⅓ of onions, cover with ⅓ of kohlrabi slices. Salt and pepper. Add ¼ of cheese mixture. Add second layer the same as first. Sprinkle flour evenly over surface. Add final layer. Pour heavy cream evenly over surface. Sprinkle remaining cheese over top.

BAKE covered at 205°C (400°F) for 45 minutes. Remove lid and bake uncovered for another 15 minutes.

 Serve with salad, roast chicken (can be roasted in the oven at the same time) and a vegetable side.

NET CARBS 9G	PROTEIN 10.8G PER SERVING

VEG

LAMB CHOPS with Minted Pea Puree and Orange Balsamic Ginger Asparagus

Serves 4 | Ready in 45 minutes

LAMB CHOPS

950g (8 small) lamb chops, room
    temperature
Sea salt for seasoning
15 mL red palm olein
3 fresh thyme sprigs
1 fresh rosemary sprig
15g (1 bulb) garlic, cut in half

MINTED PEA PUREE

300g frozen peas
10g fresh mint, chopped
75g butter
80 mL heavy cream
Salt and pepper for seasoning

ASPARAGUS

450g asparagus, washed and trimmed
Sea salt for water

BALSAMIC REDUCTION

1 orange, zested
75 mL orange juice
100 mL balsamic vinegar
15g ginger root, peeled and sliced thick

Ketogenic fine dining at its best. —CG

LAMB CHOPS

PAT lamb chops dry and season with sea salt.

PREPARE Minted Pea Puree, Asparagus, and Balsamic Reduction while lamb is curing.

HEAT palm olein in a heavy pan over medium-high heat. When the oil begins to shimmer, add the fresh rosemary and thyme to the oil. Place the sliced garlic bulb, flat side down, into the pan.

WHEN the oil is fragrant (about two minutes or so) add the lamb chops to sear. Turn chops once, cooking about three minutes on each side (for rare chops). Reserve the lovely, fragrant oil from the pan for plating.

MINTED PEA PUREE

COOK peas in water on medium-low heat until thawed. Drain. Add mint, butter, cream, and season. Using an immersion blender, blend the mixture until creamy, but the texture of peas and mint are still visible. Place the puree into the freezer immediately to preserve the colour. It will be cold, but everything else will be hot.

ASPARAGUS

PREHEAT oven to 175°C (350°F). In a deep bowl, prepare an ice bath of 50% water and 50% ice, and set aside.

BLANCH asparagus in boiling, salted water for about 2 minutes. The colour will be bright green. Remove, and place into the ice bath, then drain in a colander and place in a shallow baking dish. While lamb is searing, reheat asparagus in the oven for 5 minutes.

BALSAMIC REDUCTION

IN a small saucepan over medium-high heat, combine all ingredients and reduce until syrupy. Strain and keep warm.

PLATE the chops on a bed of the pea puree. Arrange asparagus stalks on the side. Drizzle balsamic reduction and oil from the pan around the edge. Serve and enjoy.

NET CARBS 18.5G	PROTEIN 39G PER SERVING

GF

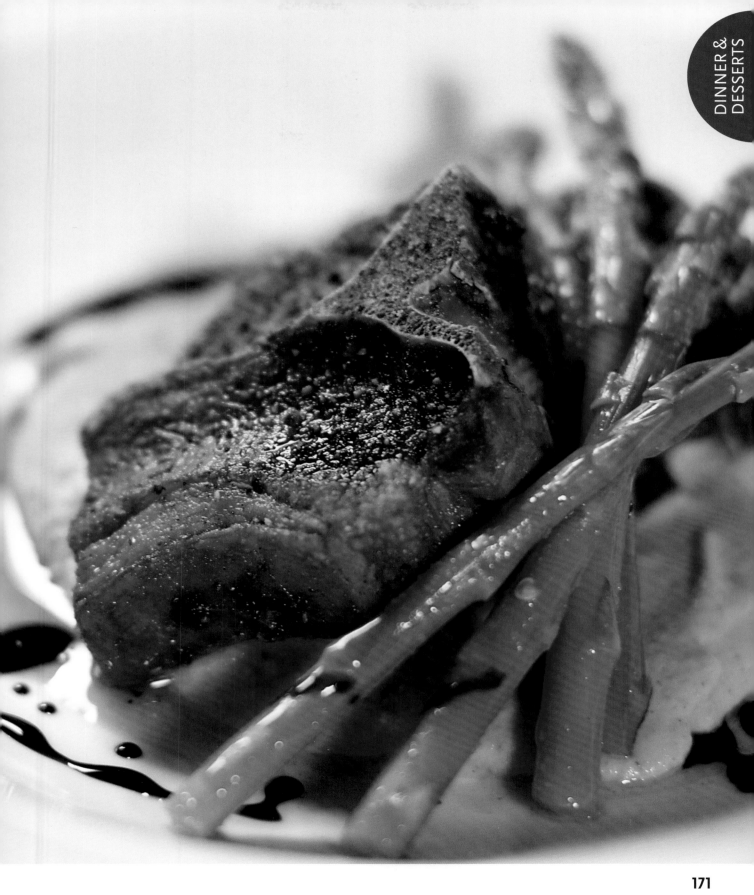

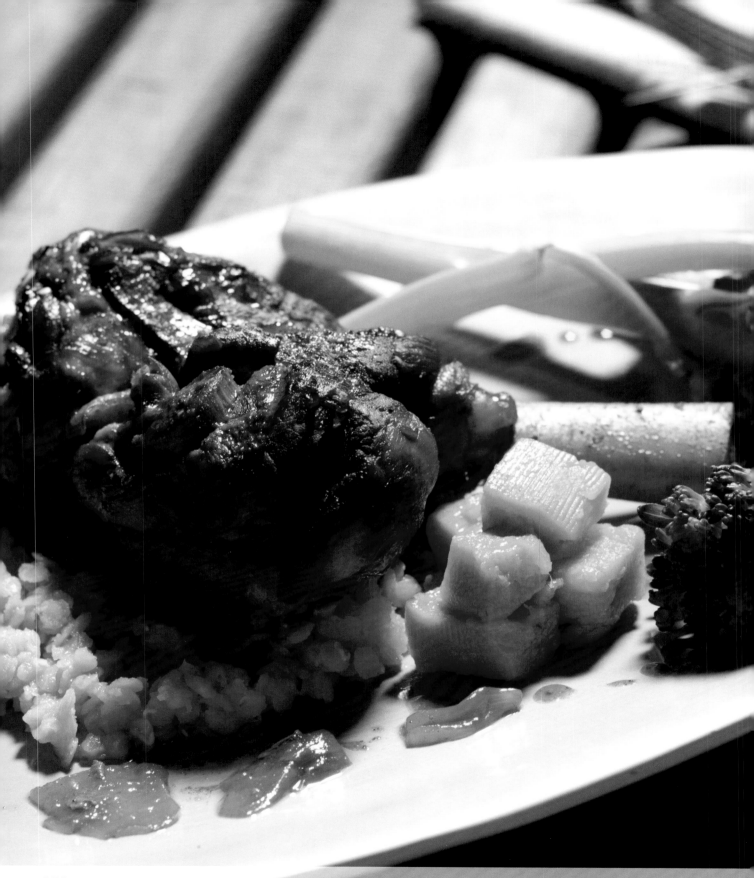

MOROCCAN LAMB BRAISE

Serves 4 | Ready in 2.5 hours

2kg (4 large) lamb shank

3 cloves

6 allspice berries

12 peppercorns

2.5 mL cardamom

2.5 mL coriander

2.5 mL cumin

5 mL turmeric

7.5 mL salt

30 mL DME™ Coconut Oil

200g onion, coarsely chopped

5g ginger, sliced

6g (3 cloves) garlic, crushed

125 mL rum

250 mL stock (chicken, beef or vegetable)

100g red lentils

500 mL water

Pinch of salt

200g green beans

I shared a meal like this with my wife in a Moroccan restaurant in Las Vegas. Lamb shank braises so nicely, with such flavour, becoming fork tender. So I decided to work up the recipe for myself. This recipe is even more flavourful than the inspiration. I hope you enjoy it as much as we did. – CG

PREHEAT oven to 150°C (300°F).

REMOVE the fell from the lamb shanks. There is no need to remove the fat or the thin membrane layer.

CRUSH the cloves, allspice, and peppercorns with a mortar and pestle. Add the salt and other spices.

MELT the coconut oil in a large pan or dutch oven over medium high heat. When the oil is shimmering, add the lamb shanks and brown on all sides. Set aside the lamb shanks on a plate to catch drippings. Turn heat down to medium-low. Add onions to the pan, along with ginger. Sauté until fragrant. Add the spices and stir. Add the garlic. Sauté until the garlic is fragrant. Add rum to deglaze pan. Reduce to half. Add chicken stock, and raise heat to bring to boil. Turn down to simmer, add lamb shanks and any drippings, cover with a tight lid, and place in oven. Braise for 2 hours. Turn shanks after one hour.

RINSE lentils under cold water. Place in a pot with water and bring to a boil. Allow to simmer for 20–25 minutes until cooked. Rinse green beans. Lightly steam for 5 minutes before plating meal.

NET CARBS 13G	PROTEIN 55.5G PER SERVING

 GF

 DAIRY FREE

MUSHROOM STUFFED BUTTERNUT SQUASH

with Walnut Sun-dried Tomato Pesto

Serves 4 | Ready in 1 hour & 15 minutes

PESTO

80g fresh basil leaves

20g sun-dried tomatoes, soaked for 30
    minutes and drained

50g raw walnuts

3g (1 clove) garlic, peeled, center removed

60 mL olive oil

SQUASH

1kg (2 small) butternut squash, halved,
    pulp discarded

30 mL butter, melted

30g shallot, chopped

5 mL butter, melted

500g white mushrooms, washed and sliced

2.5 mL dried thyme

1.5 mL dried oregano

25g Parmesan cheese, grated

Salt and pepper to taste

30g Mozzarella, grated

PREHEAT oven to 230°C (450°F).

PESTO

PULSE the basil, tomatoes, walnuts, garlic, and olive oil in a food processor or blender until smooth.

SQUASH

RUB the inside of the squash with melted butter and roast in a baking dish for 40–60 minutes until soft.

IN a frying pan, sauté the shallot in butter until soft.

ADD mushrooms, thyme, and oregano, and cook until soft. Remove from heat.

FOLD mushrooms into squash, and then add Parmesan cheese, season with salt and pepper to taste and return stuffing back to squash shells. Sprinkle each stuffed squash with Mozzarella cheese and fresh ground pepper.

BAKE squash until cheese is melted and golden brown.

PLATE half a squash per person, and add a generous dollop of the sun-dried tomato pesto just before serving.

NET CARBS 32G	PROTEIN 15.5G PER SERVING

GF   VEG

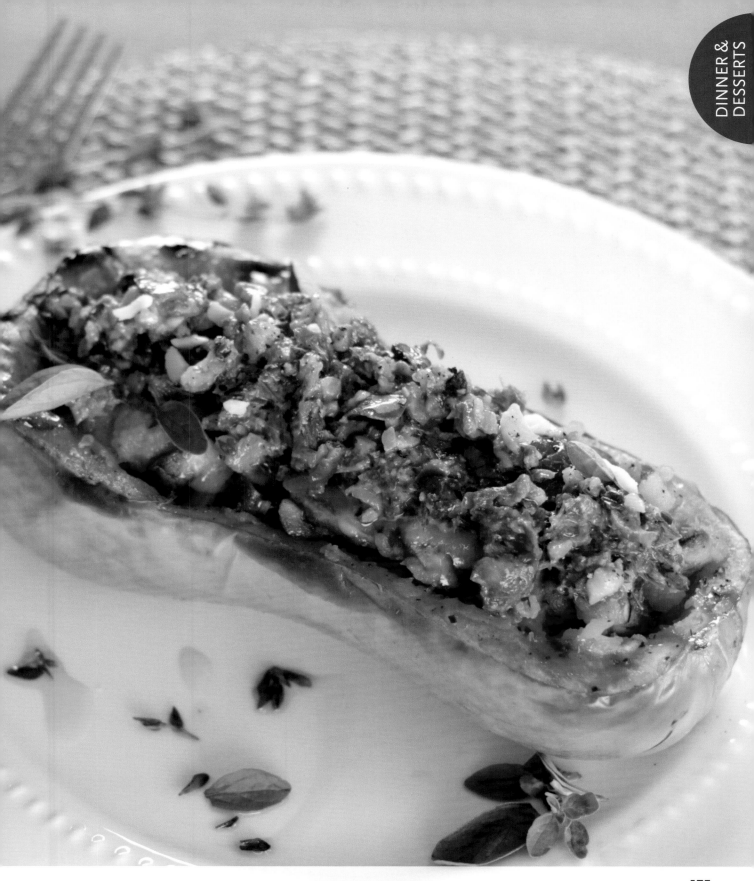

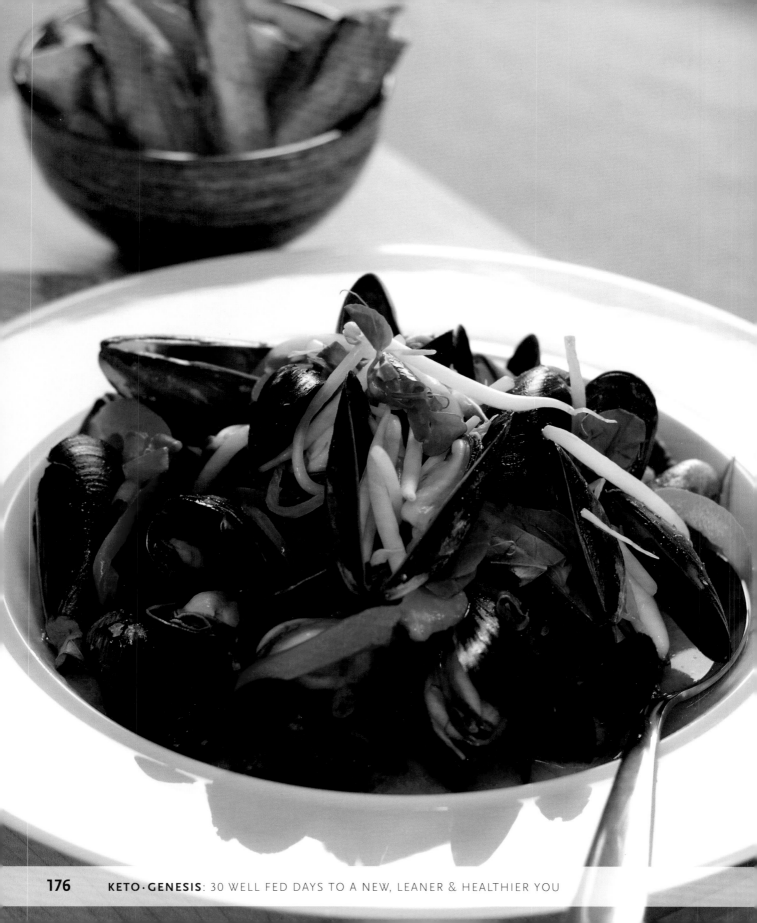

MUSSELS IN COCONUT CURRY with Yam Fries

Serves 4 | Ready in 30 minutes

MUSSELS

30 mL red palm oil or DME™ Coconut Oil,
   15 mL reserved for yams
30 mL red Thai curry paste or Indian curry
   powder
400 mL (1 can) coconut milk
100g red bell pepper, sliced
15g shallots, sliced
2 kaffir lime leaves or bay leaves
125 mL dry white wine
1kg fresh mussels, de-bearded and cleaned
50g Thai basil leaves, washed, shredded
5g green onion, chopped
125g bean sprouts, washed and patted dry

YAM FRIES

200g (2 small) yams cut into wedges
5 mL garlic powder
5 mL sea salt

This meal is made for sharing — finger food at its finest. — AT

PREHEAT oven to 220°C (425°F).

MUSSELS

IN a large sauce pan, melt red palm or coconut oil over medium heat, add curry paste or powder and stir. Slowly add coconut milk, whisking until everything is well incorporated. Add red pepper, shallot, lime leaves, and wine.

ONCE sauce is near boiling, add mussels and cover for 5–8 minutes until mussels have steamed and opened.

DISCARD any unopened mussels.

SERVE in deep bowls topped with basil, green onion, and sprouts. Spoon sauce over mussels, and discard lime leaves.

YAM FRIES

TOSS yams in red palm oil or coconut oil, and sprinkle with garlic powder and sea salt.

BAKE for 10–12 minutes until brown and crispy.

SERVE yam fries with mussels.

 Kaffir lime leaves can be found at specialty stores, and frozen for future use. Worth the extra trip, they add a brightness and depth to so many dishes.

NET CARBS 26.5G	PROTEIN 33G PER SERVING

 GF   DAIRY FREE

177

PINEAPPLE GINGER CHICKEN

Serves 4 | Ready in 40 minutes

60 mL DME™ Coconut Oil

100g ginger, cut to matchsticks

750g (1 whole) chicken, cubed, 1 ½ inch
 (ask the butcher to cut it up) or a pack of
 wings or drumettes

30g garlic, minced

125 mL Bragg's soy seasoning or coconut
 aminos

200g fresh pineapple, chunked

This is a quick and easy dish with lots of flavour I scooped from my buddy, Bill Hayer, when we were out travelling the back roads of BC together. I learned a few things from Bill, but none as tasty as this recipe. — CG

HEAT a heavy pan over medium heat. Add the coconut oil. When the oil shimmers, add the ginger, and stir until fragrant.

TURN the heat up to medium high and add the chicken to brown.

TURN the heat back down to medium, add the garlic, stir until fragrant, then deglaze with the Bragg's.

COVER and cook for about 25 minutes until the chicken pieces are done, stirring occasionally to prevent sticking. You can add a little water if you need more liquid. If there is too much liquid when done, raise the heat and cook off the excess.

ADD the fresh pineapple chunks, heat through, and serve.

 Serve alongside riced cauliflower, and for more colour, a green vegetable of your choice.

NET CARBS 13G	PROTEIN 38.8G PER SERVING

 GF   DAIRY FREE

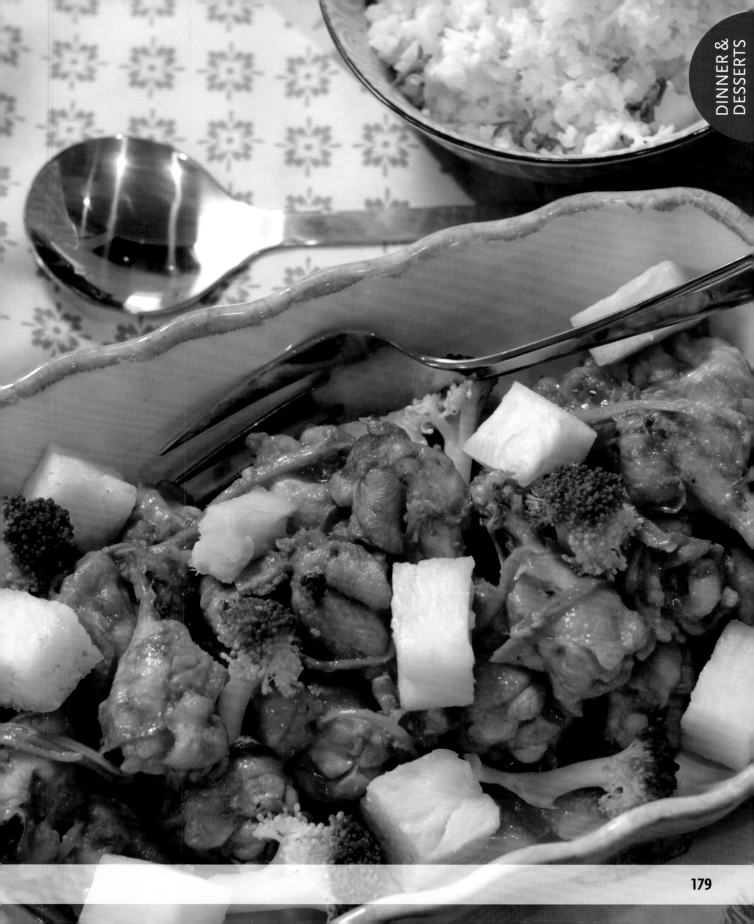

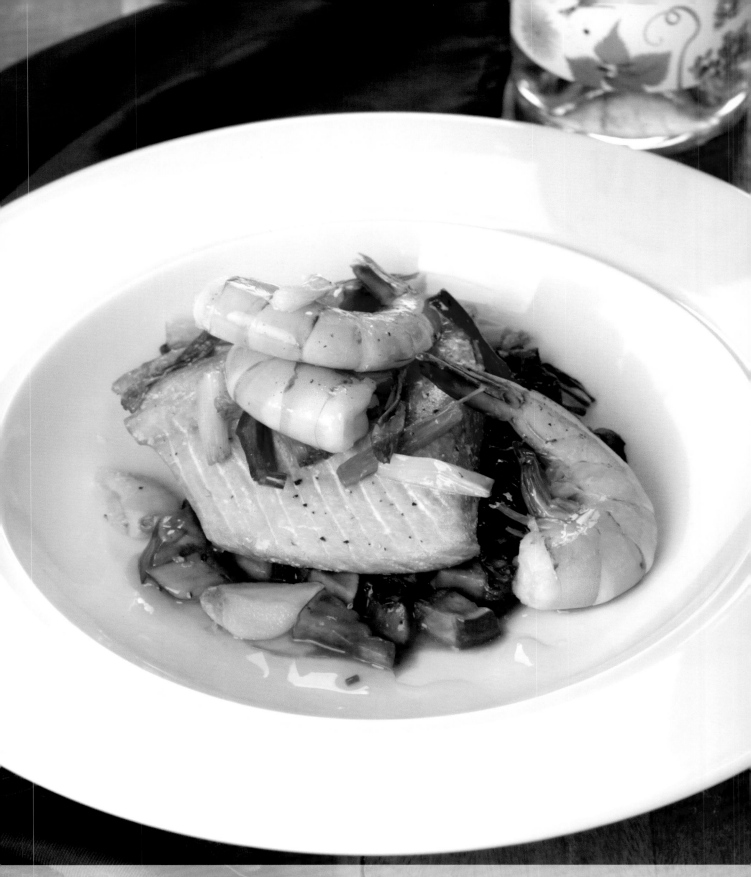

KETO·GENESIS: 30 WELL FED DAYS TO A NEW, LEANER & HEALTHIER YOU

POACHED SALMON with Portobello Mushrooms on Bed of Wilted Spinach

Serves 4 | Ready in 45 minutes

SALMON

320g wild salmon

240g prawns, in shell

60g scallions

200 mL DME™ Coconut Oil

1g Thai chili pepper

20g garlic, crushed

20g ginger, sliced

MUSHROOMS

60 mL butter

120g portobello mushrooms

125 mL white wine

140g spinach leaves

2.5 mL potato starch in 30 mL hot water

15 mL Bragg's soy seasoning

VINAIGRETTE

30 mL lime juice

30 mL rum

5 mL lime zest

1.25 mL salt

125 mL poaching oil, reserved
   after poaching salmon

PREHEAT oven to 100°C (225°F).

BRING fish to room temperature. Thaw and peel prawns.

CUT whites of scallions into 3 cm lengths. Chop greens fine.

MELT coconut oil in 25cm pan. Heat to 95°C (200°F). Fry scallion whites, Thai pepper, and crushed garlic until garlic becomes fragrant. Turn heat off, remove the flavourings from the oil and set aside on paper towel to drain. Put on separate baking tray in oven alongside fish.

ADD sliced ginger to the oil. Cool the oil back down to 50°C (120°F) measuring by thermometer. Move the ginger to one side, place the salmon and prawns in the oil. If the oil doesn't cover the salmon, add more, or place half an onion in pan face down to raise oil level. The oil should cover the prawns. Put in the oven for 25 minutes.

SAUTÉ mushrooms in 30 mL butter to thoroughly heat through over medium heat. Deglaze with wine. Stir in starch diluted in water. Raise temperature to thicken sauce. Set aside and keep warm.

HEAT 30 mL butter in pan. Sauté spinach leaves until lightly wilted. Stir in Bragg's. Serve mushrooms on bed of wilted spinach.

LIFT salmon and prawns out of oil and place on warmed plates to serve. Reserve 125 mL poaching oil for vinaigrette. Combine oil with vinaigrette ingredients and whisk together. Arrange spinach and mushrooms. Dress salmon with vinaigrette, garnish with scallion greens, and serve. Serve scallion whites and garlic on side. The Thai chili is for the adventurous types at the dinner party.

 Poaching in oil is an amazing way to prepare fish. You can replace the salmon with halibut or other firm fleshed fish. The DME™ Coconut Oil is expensive, but the coconut flavour is more intense than other oils, which translates to a better tasting dish.

NET CARBS 6.5G	PROTEIN 32.2G PER SERVING

GF

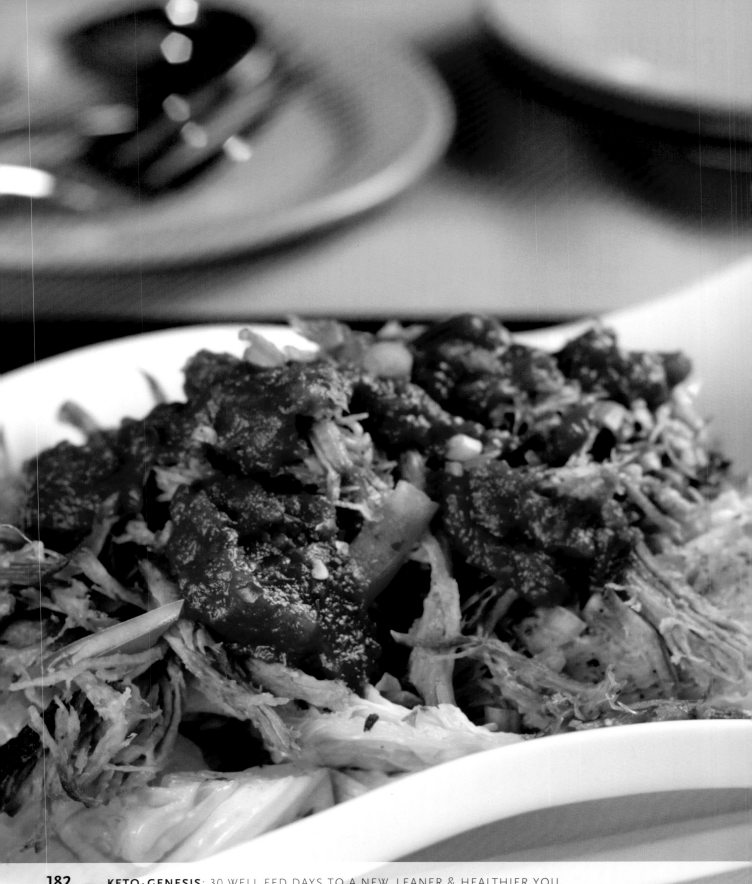

PULLED PORK on Braised Cabbage

Serves 8 | Ready in 2 hours 20 minutes

PULLED PORK

3kg pork shoulder

10 mL salt

2.5 mL black pepper, fresh ground

400g onions, chopped coarsely

30g garlic, crushed

5 mL chili powder

5 mL cumin

5 mL cardamom

15 mL coriander

15 mL paprika

30 mL DME™ Coconut Oil

60 mL whiskey

125 mL stock, vegetable or beef

60 mL molasses

CABBAGE

1kg cabbage

1.25 mL salt

60 mL stock, vegetable or beef

60 mL camelina oil

PULLED PORK

PREHEAT oven to 160°C (325°F).

DRY the pork, and salt with 5 mL of salt. Season with pepper.

CHOP onions coarsely. Peel and crush the garlic with the flat of a chef's knife. Mix spices and remaining salt together in a bowl.

HEAT coconut oil in a 30cm dutch oven or skillet with tight fitting lid. When it shimmers, sear pork on all sides, about 3 minutes per side. Remove pork, and set it aside on a plate to catch the drippings.

TURN the heat down to medium low. Add onions to the pan, and sauté until soft. Add crushed garlic and spices. Sauté until fragrant. Deglaze pan with the whiskey. Add stock, then the molasses, and bring to boil to meld flavours.

TURN heat down to simmer, then add the pork and the collected juices to the pan. Place a piece of parchment paper (cut to slightly larger than the lid) under the lid to form a tight seal. Place on the lower rack in the oven. After one hour, turn pork. Braise for another hour, or until the pork can be pulled apart with a fork.

LIFT pork out and set aside to cool. When cooled, peel it apart with two forks.

STRAIN the liquid, pressing on the solid bits to extract the liquid. Discard the solids and pour off the fat. Add the sauce to the pulled pork to moisten it.

CABBAGE

PEEL outer leaves off of the cabbage and discard. Cut cabbage in half and core. Cut into 1 cm thick slices. Place slices in baking dish. Salt. Add stock to the baking dish, and drizzle the cabbage with camelina oil. Cover the dish with foil, and place into the oven alongside the pork for two hours, or until the cabbage is soft.

SERVE the pulled pork on top of the cabbage bed. Top with Barbeque Sauce (page 215).

NET CARBS 12G	PROTEIN 66G PER SERVING

 DAIRY FREE

RED LENTIL CURRY

Serves 6 | Ready in 50 minutes

200g red lentils

15 mL DME™ Coconut Oil

100g onion, chopped coarse

5g ginger, sliced

30 mL Madras Curry Paste (page 219)

60 mL rum

500 mL vegetable stock

400g daikon, cubed

200g carrots, chopped

30 mL Alpha Balance™ Oil

20g parsley, chopped fine

This is a great vegan curry. Just make it for the omnivores, along with Christel's Nut Falafel (page 154), and don't say anything. The compliments will arrive on their own. —CG

WASH lentils in colander to clean thoroughly.

HEAT coconut oil in pan until it shimmers. Add onions and ginger, and sauté until fragrant. Add curry paste and heat through. Deglaze pan with rum. Add stock, daikon, carrots, and lentils. Bring to a boil, then turn down to simmer and cover with a lid. Simmer for 20–25 minutes until the daikon is soft enough to pierce with a fork, and the lentils are soft. Stir in the Alpha Balance™ Oil and simmer for another two minutes to meld flavours. Garnish with parsley.

NET CARBS 21G	PROTEIN 10G PER SERVING

GF VEGAN DAIRY FREE VEG

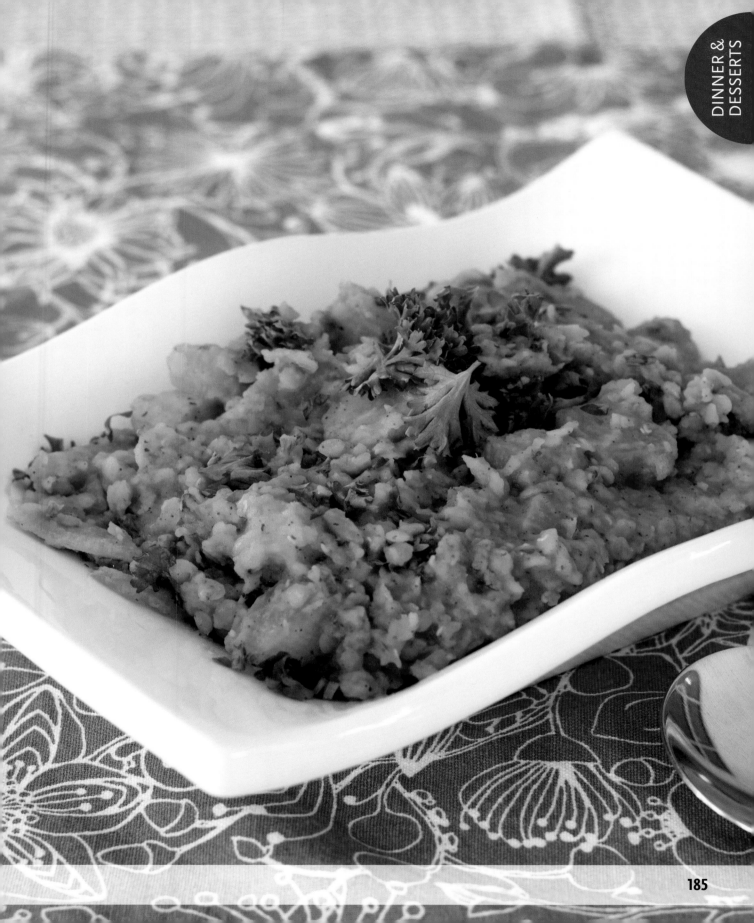

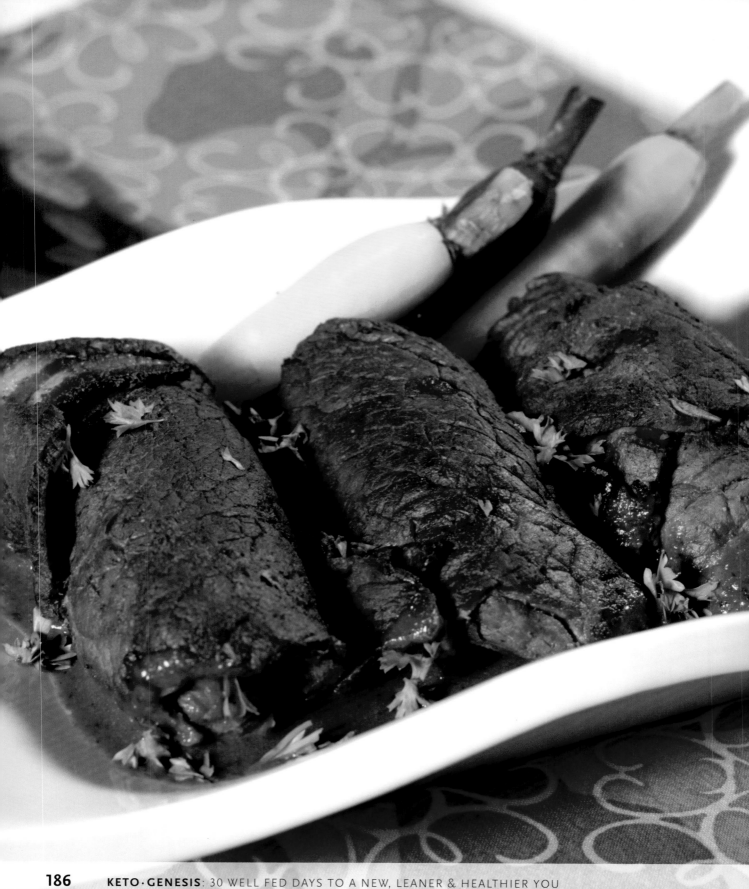

BRAISED ROULADEN

Serves 6 | Ready in 2 hours 45 minutes

6 beef rouladen (inside round, sliced thin)
60 mL mustard
Salt and pepper to taste
6 bacon strips
6 dill pickles
15 mL DME™ Coconut Oil

100g onion, diced large
100g carrots, peeled
75g celery stalks
12g (4 cloves) garlic, crushed
125 mL stock, beef or vegetable
125 mL red wine
60 mL pickle juice
6 toothpicks
125 mL sour cream (optional)

This was our traditional Sunday meal growing up. We've made this dish for friends many times, and first-timers are always surprised that rouladen are available at the meat counter. Even check-out clerks have asked me, "what are you going to make with that?" Now you know too! – CG

PREHEAT oven to 160°C (325°F).

SPREAD the rouladen out on the work surface. Apply a thin coating of mustard to each, then salt and pepper. Place bacon strip on top, then roll beef and bacon around the dill pickle. Use the toothpick to secure. Use paper towels to dry the rouladen for a better sear.

HEAT the coconut oil in a dutch oven until shimmering. Brown the rouladen on 4 sides. Remove from the pan onto a plate. Add the onions and carrots to the pan and brown lightly. Add crushed garlic and celery stalk. Sauté until fragrant. Deglaze pan with red wine. Add stock and pickle juice and bring to boil to combine flavours.

TURN down to simmer. Add the rouladen back into the pan along with collected juices. Cover with parchment paper and lid to form a tight seal, and place into oven for 2½ hours. Turn rouladen after 1 hour.

WHEN the meat is done to the point of falling apart, remove from oven. Using tongs, put rouladen on a plate and cover with foil to keep warm. Separate the fat and remove the vegetables. Reduce the sauce by boiling. Sour cream may be added to thicken. Salt and pepper to taste. Serve sauce separately.

SERVE with salad, roasted root vegetables and broccoli.

 This recipe may be transferred from a pan to a covered clay baking dish for the oven, or it can be made in the slow cooker as well. The braised vegetables can be puréed back into the reduced sauce to provide additional body. This is also an easy recipe to double up, and most large dutch ovens or clay bakers can hold 12 rouladen.

NET CARBS 5G	PROTEIN 26G PER SERVING

 GF   DAIRY FREE

SASHIMI AND JICAMA RICE BOWL with Sesame Miso Dressing

Serves 2 (or 4 as a side dish or appetizer) | Ready in 35 minutes

600g (1 medium) jicama, peeled and pulsed
    until rice-like in a food processor
300g avocados, ripe and sliced
400g sashimi-grade wild salmon, tuna, or
    tuna belly
100g carrots, shredded
50g broccoli sprouts
75g red bell pepper, diced
5g white sesame seeds
5g black sesame seeds
1 sheet of nori, shredded

DRESSING

60 mL sesame oil
125 mL rice wine vinegar
15 mL fresh lemon or lime juice
15 mL miso paste
1.5 mL prepared wasabi
1.5 mL Bragg's or other soy sauce substitute

This meal is inspired by all of the beautiful sushi we have here on the West Coast. —AT

PREPARE the dressing by blending all ingredients in a blender or small food processor.

PLACE your jicama rice in bowls, about 300g per bowl.

ADD broccoli sprouts, carrots, and red pepper, and top with avocado.

POUR dressing over vegetables.

PLACE your fish on a cutting board, and using a sharp knife, cut into ½-inch strips.

TOP bowls with fish, sesame seeds, and shredded nori. Enjoy!

NET CARBS 13.5G	PROTEIN 25.7G PER SERVING

 GF   DAIRY FREE

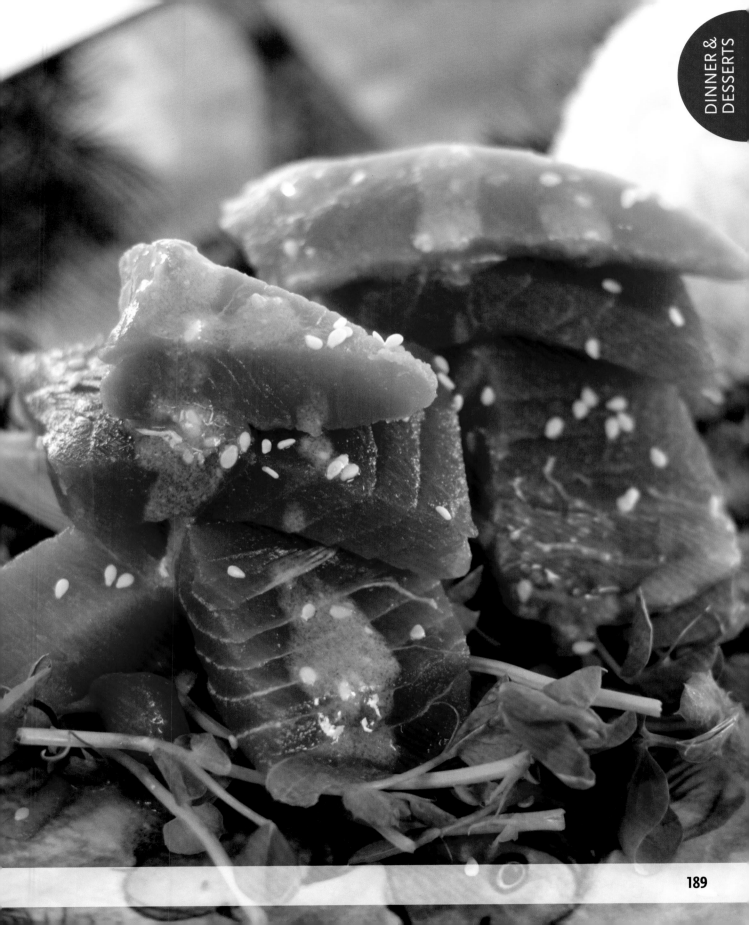

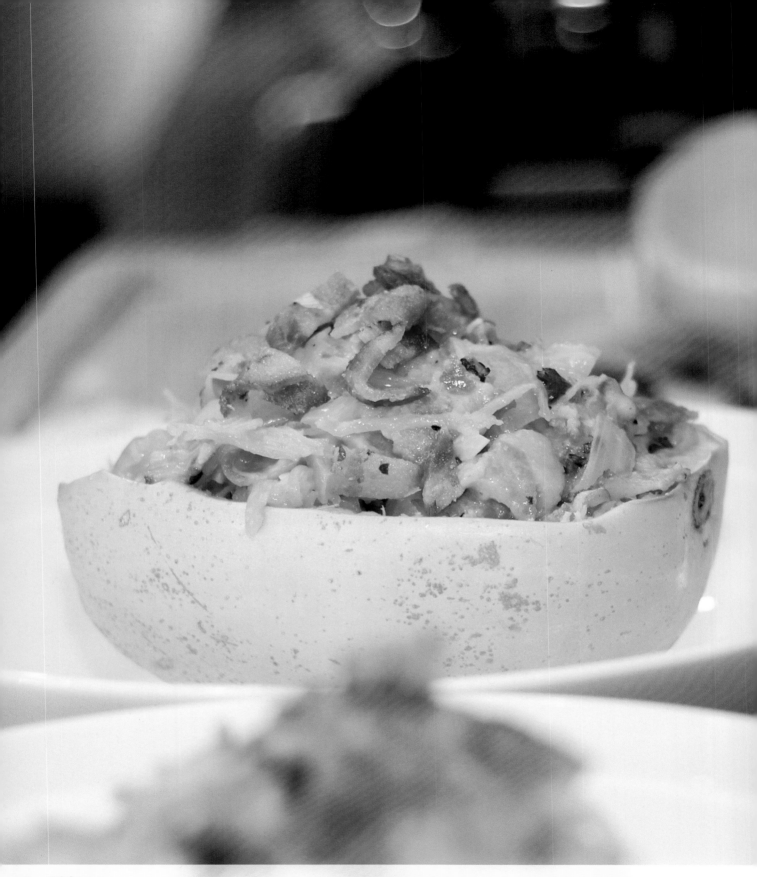

SPAGHETTI SQUASH CARBONARA

Serves 8 | Ready in 55 minutes

1500g spaghetti squash

250 mL heavy (whipping) cream

200g bacon, cut into 1cm pieces

100g onion, diced

10g (3 medium cloves) garlic, minced

60 mL dry white wine

3 eggs

100g Parmesan cheese, finely grated

2.5 mL salt (or to taste)

2.5 mL white or black ground pepper

1.25 mL nutmeg

2.5 mL parsley

2.5 mL Worcester sauce

PREHEAT oven to 175°C (350°F).

CUT spaghetti squash in half lengthwise. Trim off the stem and remove seeds. Place each half cut-side down in a baking dish. Add ½ inch water and cover with foil. Bake for 40 minutes until tender. Cool. Using a fork, scrape squash from its shell and separate the strands. They should look like spaghetti. This step can be done ahead of time.

IN the meantime, place the cream in a small pot and reduce to half over low heat. Stir regularly to prevent burning. A little browning is alright, and will add to the complexity of the flavour. This will take about 30 minutes.

USING a large heavy sauce pan, cook the bacon. When it is about ½ cooked, add onions and continue until almost done. Add garlic and sauté until fragrant. Deglaze with white wine, and reduce to half. Add the spaghetti squash and heat through.

IN a small bowl, whisk together eggs, grated Parmesan, and seasonings.

TAKE the squash mixture off the heat. Pour the reduced cream over the squash, toss, then add the cheese mixture. Toss again until the squash is evenly coated. Serve immediately.

 The heat retained in the squash will cook the egg mixture without overheating it.

NET CARBS 14.2G	PROTEIN 13.2G PER SERVING

GF

TACO SALAD

Serves 2 | Cook time 30 min

200g ground beef
30 mL DME™ Coconut Oil
50g onion, diced fine
10g (3 medium cloves) garlic, minced
5 mL salt
60 mL chili powder
60 mL water

100g mixed greens
100g daikon, sliced thin
50g aged Cheddar, grated
200g avocado
100g bell pepper
125g tomato
50g onion
125 mL salsa
125 mL sour cream

HEAT the oil in a medium pan over medium heat. Add the ground beef. As it begins to brown, add the onions, then the garlic and salt. When brown, add the chili powder and the water, stir to mix thoroughly. Cook until the liquid has evaporated, stirring occasionally.

ARRANGE the mixed greens in a deep dish, layer the daikon radish, then the meat, cheese, and vegetables. Top with salsa and sour cream.

 The daikon provides the snap that usually comes from the corn chips. Make sure to find a natural sour cream without starch additions, or make your own clabbered cream (see tip on page 59).

NET CARBS 17.5G	PROTEIN 36G PER SERVING

GF

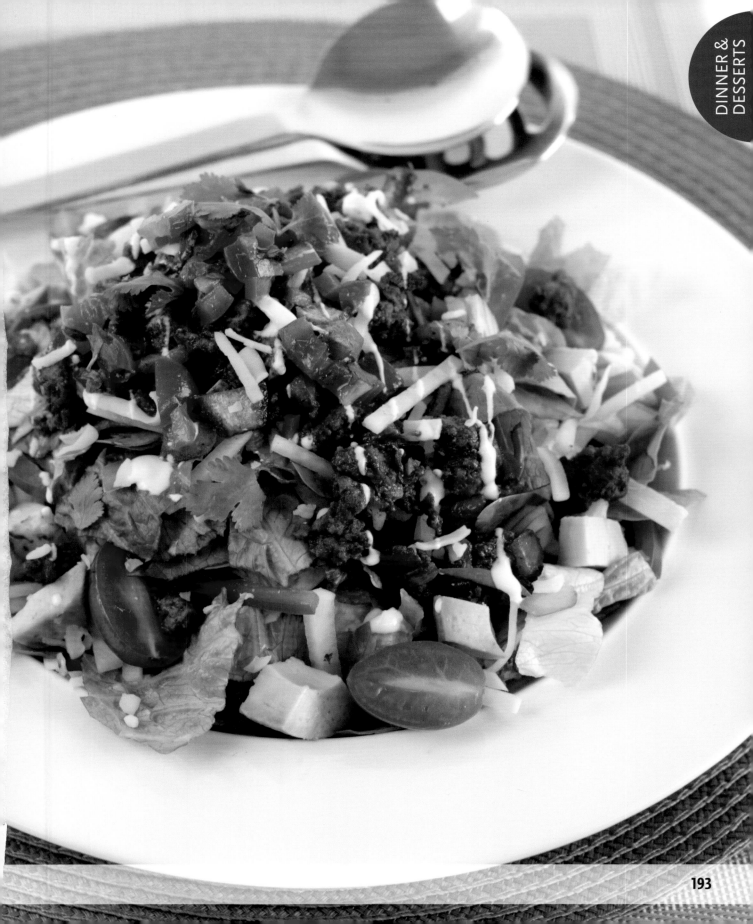

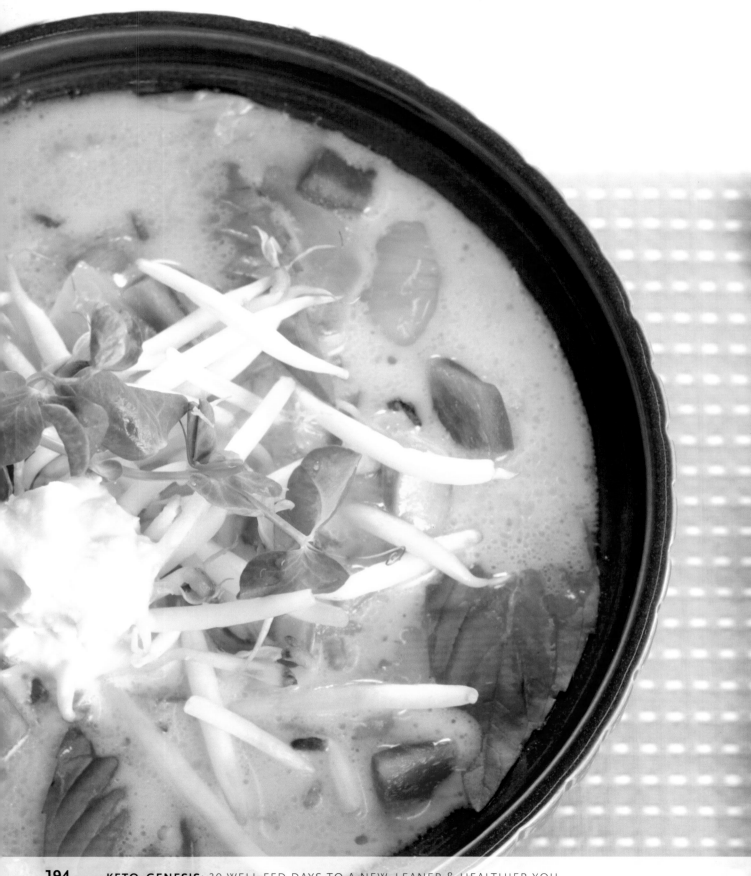

THAI CHICKEN CURRY

Serves 4 | Ready in 45 minutes

30g DME™ Coconut Oil

450g chicken wings

150g Napa cabbage, shredded

100g onion, trimmed and cut in quarters

100g carrots, diced small

150g daikon, diced small

10g (3 medium cloves) garlic, sliced

40g Thai Curry Paste (page 218)

500 mL chicken stock

10 mL lime juice

½ lime, zested

7.5 mL salt

150g chicken thighs, boneless, skinless,
    diced 1cm

250 mL coconut milk, full fat

20g fresh basil, shredded

100g red bell pepper, diced

300g mung bean sprouts

LIME COCONUT CREAM

100 mL coconut cream

½ lime, zested

5 mL lime juice

The lime coconut cream is an inspiration. It's amazing how different the flavour is, even though the recipe already contains both coconut and lime. —CG

HEAT coconut oil in 12-inch dutch oven over medium high heat. Pat chicken wings dry, and pan sear both sides. Use splatter screen to prevent oil splatters. Set aside.

TURN heat down to medium low heat. Add the Napa cabbage, onions, carrots, and daikon to the pan and sauté. The moisture from the vegetables should loosen any brown bits left over from the chicken. When the onions start to become soft, add the sliced garlic and sauté until fragrant. Add the curry paste, and combine thoroughly. Add the stock to deglaze. Add the lime juice, zest, and the salt, turn the heat up and bring to a brief boil to meld flavours. Turn back down to medium low heat, stir in the diced chicken thighs, and add the reserved wings. Stir in the coconut milk and add the shredded basil. Cover with a lid and simmer until the chicken pieces are done, about 25 minutes. If you prefer the curry to be more liquid, add some water before simmering. Add the red pepper, and heat through. Salt to taste.

WHILE the curry is simmering, add lime zest to coconut cream and whisk for about 5 minutes. Fold in lime juice after whipping.

RINSE bean sprouts.

SERVE the curry in a rimmed soup bowl. Dress with mung bean sprouts and a dollop of coconut lime cream.

 For the coconut cream, buy full fat coconut milk, refrigerate it, and then scoop out only the thick white cream. Use the water in a Piña Colada Super Green Smoothie (page 55).

NET CARBS 17G	PROTEIN 26.3G PER SERVING

 GF   DAIRY FREE

195

THREE CHEESE SOUP with Butternut Squash Croutons

Serves 4 | Ready in 50 minutes

CROUTONS

125g butternut squash, cubed
15 mL red palm oil
5 mL sea salt
1.5 mL smoked paprika

SOUP

30 mL butter, red palm oil, or camelina oil
250g sweet onion, diced
150g celery, diced
150g carrots, diced
2.5 mL sea salt
30g arrowroot starch
1L chicken, beef, or vegetable broth
   preferably homemade
6g (2 cloves) garlic, crushed
1 bay leaf
250 mL heavy (whipping) cream
1.5 mL crushed red pepper flakes
225g shredded cheese (a mix of Cheddar,
   Gruyère, Queso Fresco or Haloumi will
   melt well)
60 mL dry white wine
Salt and pepper to taste

That's right — cheese soup. A lovely treat for your well earned weekend. — AT

CROUTONS

PREHEAT oven to 220°C (425°F).

TOSS butternut squash in oil and seasoning. Bake for 20 minutes, until crispy, turning every 5 minutes to ensure even cooking.

REMOVE squash and drain on paper towel uncovered.

SOUP

IN a large sauce pan, melt butter or heat oil over medium heat. Add onion, celery, carrot, and salt, and sauté for 5 minutes. Slowly add flour, stirring to prevent lumps, for 3 minutes.

GRADUALLY add stock and bring to a gentle boil. Reduce and add garlic, bay leaf and red pepper. Simmer for twenty minutes until vegetables are soft. Remove bay leaf, and remove pot from heat. Add the whipping cream.

USING an immersion blender, blend the vegetables into the broth until smooth.

ADD the cheese, a little at a time, whisking until melted.

ADD wine and return to low heat until well blended and warm enough to serve.

DIVIDE into bowls and top with Butternut Croutons.

 You may use all of one kind of cheese, Cheddar being the easiest to find.

NET CARBS 21.8G	PROTEIN 18.9G PER SERVING

GF   VEG

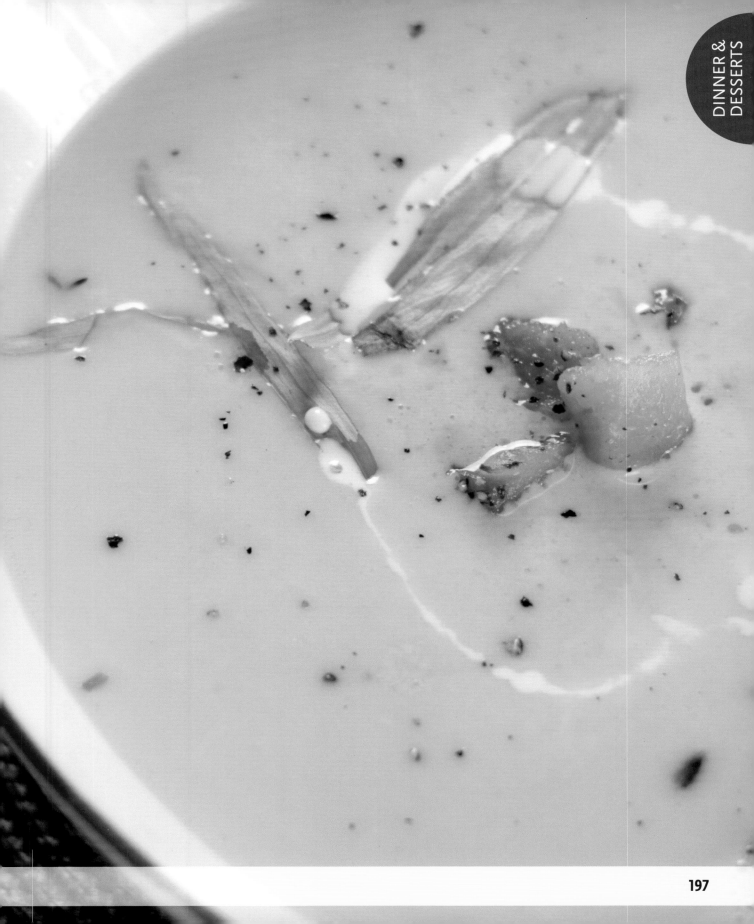

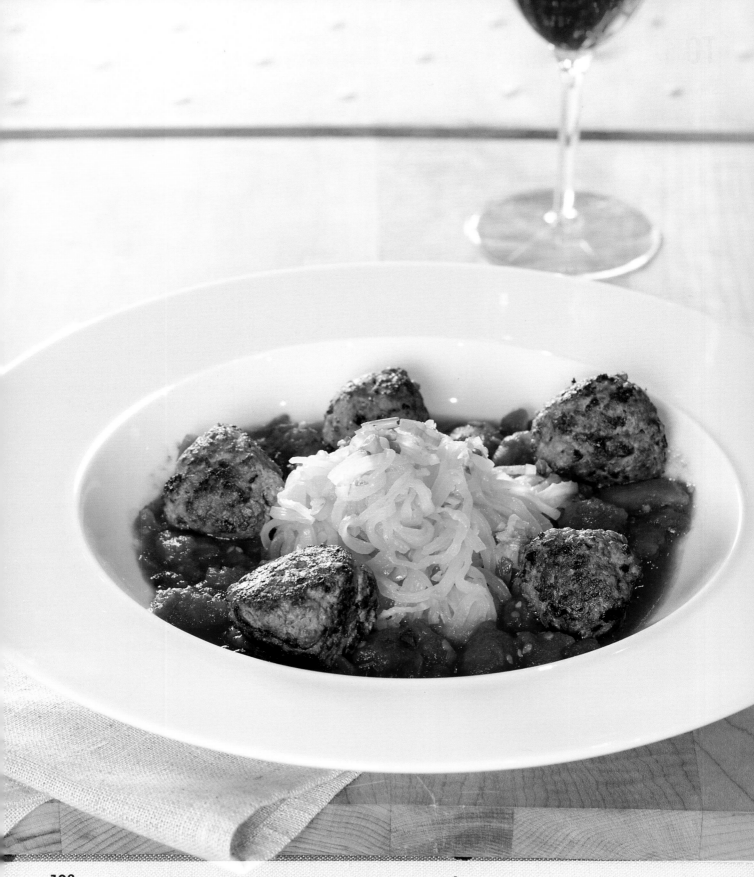

TOMATO AND MEATBALLS over Daikon Radish

Serves 4 (Makes 12 (1½-inch) meatballs) | Ready in 45 minutes

TOMATO SAUCE

30 mL DME™ Coconut Oil

50g onion, diced

20g mushrooms, sliced

10g garlic, minced

400 mL canned tomatoes, diced

125 mL red wine

1.25 mL rosemary, ground

1.25 mL oregano, ground

5 mL maple syrup

1.25 mL thyme, ground

1.25 mL basil, ground

MEATBALLS

300g ground beef

30g onions, diced

10g garlic, minced

5 mL parsley, ground

5 mL oregano, ground

2.5 mL rosemary, ground

5 mL salt

2.5 mL black pepper, coarse ground

5 mL Tabasco sauce

1 egg

DAIKON BED

400g daikon, julienned

60 mL chicken stock

30g butter

As a child, I hated "replacement food." Carob was not a replacement for chocolate, and honey ice cream was not a replacement for vanilla. So daikon isn't a replacement for noodles. But it is a good accompaniment for tomato and meatballs. And it's low in carbohydrates, which makes a meal with tomato sauce possible. — CG

SAUCE

SAUTÉ the onions in the coconut oil over medium low heat until soft. Add the mushrooms, and sauté until they give up their liquid. Add the garlic and sauté until fragrant. Deglaze the pan with the wine, add tomatoes, herbs, and maple syrup. Bring to a brief boil, then turn down the heat and let simmer uncovered over low heat while preparing the rest of the meal. Stir occasionally.

MEATBALLS

PREHEAT the oven to 205°C (400°F). Mix all the ingredients together by hand in a medium bowl. Form the meatballs and set them on parchment paper on a baking sheet. Bake 30 minutes.

DAIKON

PLACE daikon in an open sauce pan with stock and butter. Bring to a boil, then lower heat to simmer, until liquid is mostly reduced. Toss daikon in remaining mixture to coat.

 TIP Sautéing the daikon takes off the sharp radish edge, leaving it mellow and al dente.

NET CARBS 16G	PROTEIN 24G PER SERVING

GF

ULTIMATE THAI STIR FRY

Serves 4 | Ready in 25 minutes

300g (2 large) chicken breasts, sliced
    diagonally
9g (3 small cloves) garlic
15 mL Bragg's soy seasoning
    plus 60 mL for stir fry
85 mL camelina oil
200g broccoli florets
250g carrots, sliced into ribbons
    using the peeler
75g onion, halved and sliced
1.25 mL honey
15 mL oyster sauce
2 eggs, beaten
100g bean sprouts
15g roasted peanuts, crushed
25g green onions, chopped

This recipe is inspired by my favourite Thai restaurant on Cambie Street in Vancouver, BC. — AT

MARINATE chicken in garlic and 15 mL of Bragg's sauce for thirty minutes before cooking.

IN a wok, heat the camelina oil on medium heat, and add chicken, cooking until almost done. Remove and set aside. Set aside wok as you will need it shortly.

IN a separate pot, steam broccoli for two minutes and rinse under cold water.

SAUTÉ carrot ribbons, onions, oyster sauce, soy sauce and honey until soft.

ADD chicken back to pan, add eggs, and stir gently.

FOLD in broccoli and cook for another minute.

SERVE immediately topped with sprouts, peanuts, and green onions.

NET CARBS 13.2G	PROTEIN 38.8G PER SERVING

 GF   DAIRY FREE

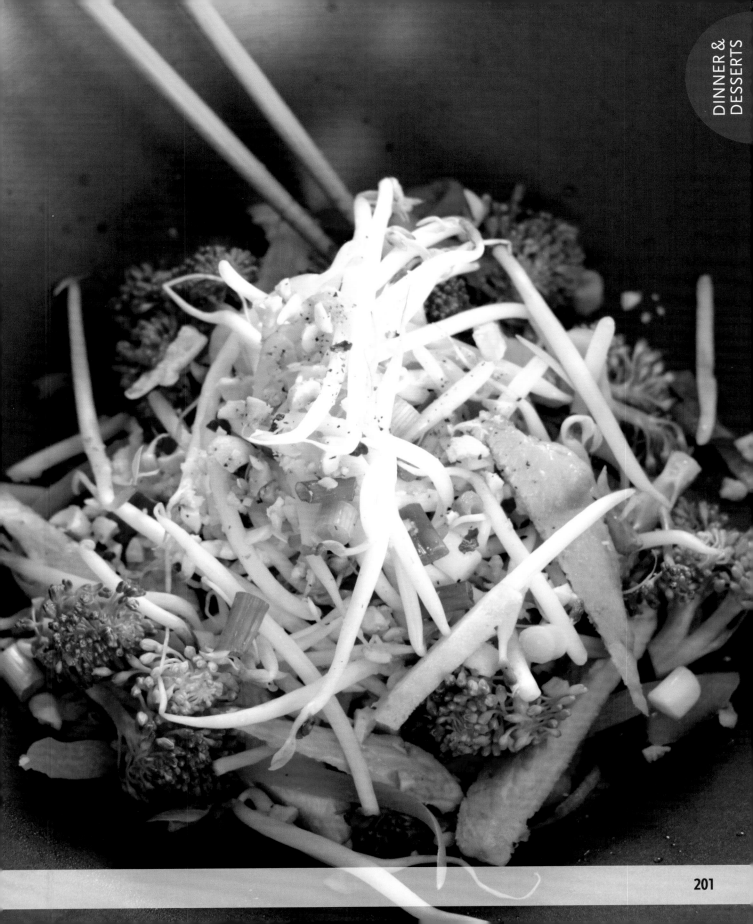

ANGEL FOOD CAKE

Serves 10 | Ready in 45 minutes

250g egg white (room temperature)
1.25 mL vanilla
1.25 mL almond flavouring
15 mL cold water (or ½ water and
    ½ lemon juice)
2.5 mL cream of tartar
60g all-purpose flour
30g white sugar
1.25 mL salt

This is the only recipe in which we use white sugar. There's something about coconut sugar that causes the egg whites to fall. We're still trying other options. – CG

PREHEAT oven to 175°C (350°F).

IN large bowl, whip egg whites ¼ of the way and then add almond, vanilla, and water. About halfway through beating the eggs, gradually add cream of tartar while continuing to beat. Beat until stiff.

IN a medium bowl, combine flour, sugar, and salt. Put this mixture through sifter 5 times.

SIFT dry ingredients over egg whites 1/3 at a time and fold after each addition until smooth.

SPREAD batter into a greased bundt or angel food cake pan.

BAKE for 20–25 minutes, until golden. Cool completely.

 Best served with fresh fruit and whipping cream.

NET CARBS 7.7G	PROTEIN 3.4G PER SERVING

VEG   DAIRY FREE

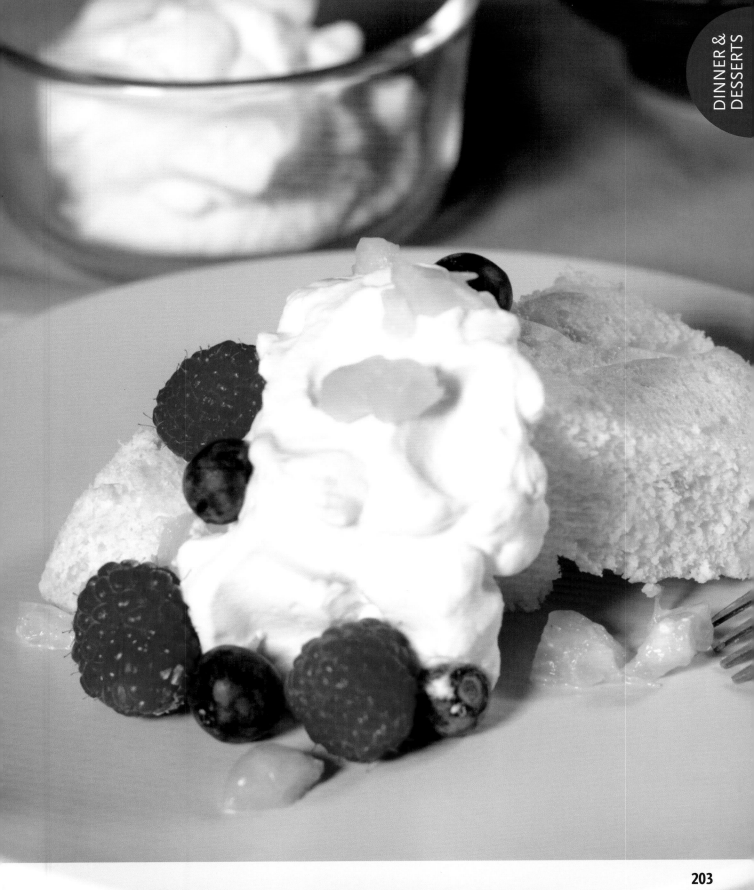

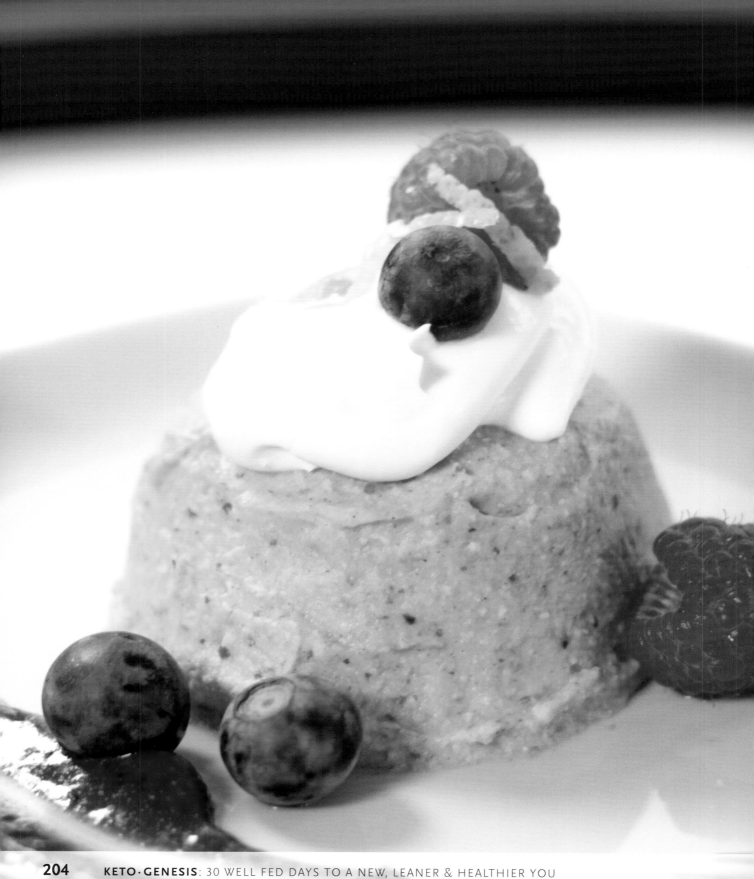

HAZELNUT SQUASH DESSERT

Serves 8 | Ready in 45 minutes

400g butternut squash

350g Granny Smith apples, peeled, cored & quartered

60 mL red palm olein for baking

120g hazelnuts

20g flaxseed

1.5 mL coriander seed

1.5 mL nutmeg

2.5 mL cardamom

5 mL cinnamon

5 mL salt

45 mL Alpha Balance™ Oil

Now that we're empty nesters, some produce, gourds in particular, are too much to use in a single meal. So we've come up with some interesting alternatives to make use of what we have. This recipe refrigerates well, and can even be frozen, to be thawed at a later time. —CG

PREHEAT oven to 205°C (400°F.)

CUT the butternut squash in half, then seed, peel, and cube into 1cm cubes. Peel, quarter and core the apples. Place the squash and apple quarters onto a baking sheet greased with red palm olein, and place into the oven for 20 minutes or until soft.

WHEN soft, put the squash and apple into a food processor.

GRIND the nuts and the flaxseed in a grinder. Add to the food processor, along with the spices, salt, and Alpha Balance™ Oil, and purée.

LET cool to room temperature and serve with whipped vanilla cream or whipped coconut cream.

TIP You can use this same mixture to make the Hazelnut Squash Fritters (page 103).

NET CARBS 11G	PROTEIN 3.3G PER SERVING

 GF   VEGAN   DAIRY FREE   VEG

ICED CHOCOLATE CHILI BROWNIES

Serves 12 | Ready in 35 minutes

330g black beans, cooked and rinsed
80g coconut sugar
120g cocoa powder
5 mL baking powder
2.5 mL cayenne pepper
2 eggs
10 mL vanilla
125 mL DME™ Coconut Oil, melted

A melt-in-your-mouth delicious treat with a subtle kick of heat.
– AT

PREHEAT oven to 175°C (350°F), and grease an 8"x 10" baking pan with a small amount of coconut oil.

ADD your first five ingredients to a food processor until well blended.

ADD remaining ingredients and blend until smooth – a bit of texture is ok. Smooth batter evenly over baking pan. It should be thick, but will spread easily.

BAKE for 25–30 minutes, until a toothpick comes out clean.

ALLOW to sit for 5 minutes before serving.

TOP brownies with a spoonful of chocolate icing (recipe follows), or simply enjoy on their own.

NET CARBS 12G	PROTEIN 4.6G PER SERVING

 GF   VEG   DAIRY FREE

CHOCOLATE ICING

Serves 16 | Ready in 5 minutes

250 mL DME™ Coconut Oil, melted
60g cocoa powder
1.25 mL cinnamon
30 mL maple syrup
5 mL vanilla

MIX all ingredients until smooth.

TOP your brownies or refrigerate and save for later.

 TIP If keeping in fridge, allow to sit out at room temperature to soften before using. Because of coconut oil, icing will harden when refrigerated.

NET CARBS 2.5G	PROTEIN .75G PER 15 ML SERVING

 GF   VEGAN DAIRY FREE VEG

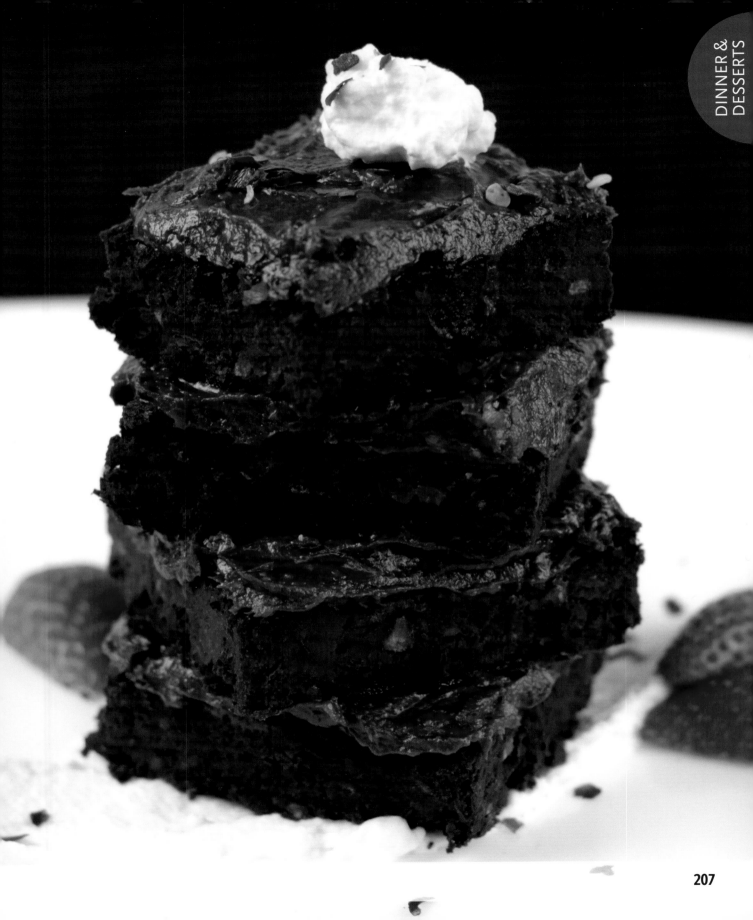

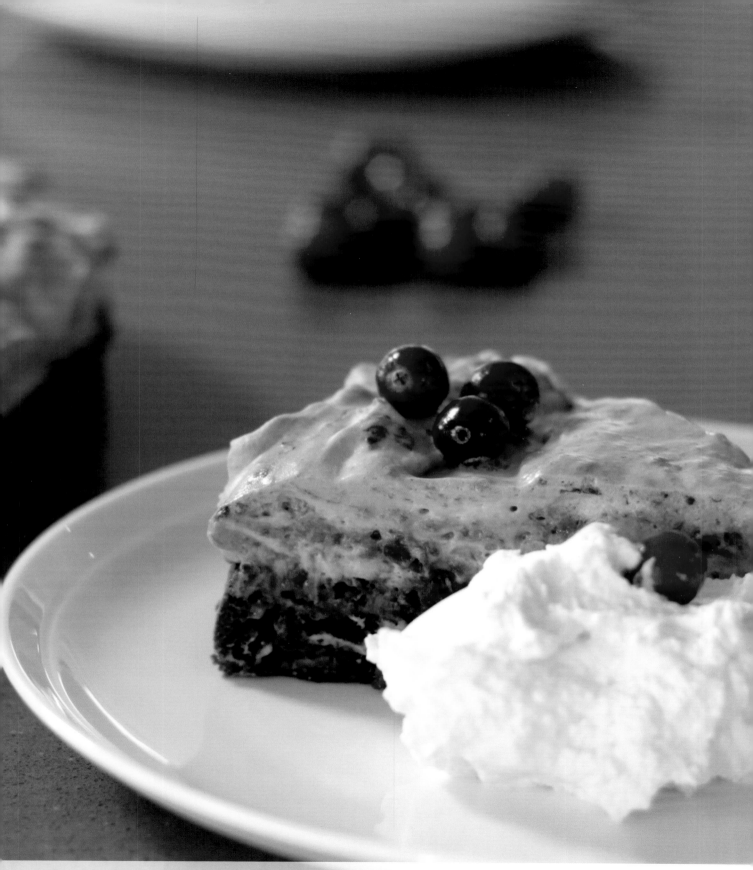

JAEGER TORTE

Serves 12 | Ready in 4–5 hours

BASE

3 eggs, separated
125g butter, melted and cooled
50g coconut sugar
125g hazelnuts, ground
30g cocoa
5 mL baking powder
5 mL vanilla

TOPPING

Dash of salt
115g coconut sugar
90 mL water + 25 mL water
170g cranberries
3.5g gelatin
250 mL heavy (whipping) cream

Nobody is better at combining sugar, fat, and flour than the Germans. Seriously. We've cut back on the sugar, eliminated the flour, and it still tastes heavenly. – CG

BASE

PREHEAT oven to 175°C (350°F).

COMBINE butter, sugar, and egg yolks. Add hazelnuts, cocoa, baking powder and salt, and mix well. In a separate bowl, mix egg whites until stiff. Gently fold egg whites into the base mixture. Smooth into a 10-inch spring form pan.

BAKE for 20 minutes, checking after 12 minutes, then cool completely.

TOPPING

DISSOLVE the salt and sugar in 90 mL of water, bringing to boil in a non-reactive pot over high heat. Stir in the cranberries. Return to boil. Lower heat to medium and simmer until slightly thickened and ⅔ of the cranberries have popped open – about 5 minutes.

MEANWHILE, dissolve gelatin in 25 mL of water.

TRANSFER cranberries to non-reactive bowl. Stir in dissolved gelatin mixture. Refrigerate for 15 minutes.

WHIP 250 mL of heavy cream until firm. Fold into cold cranberry sauce. Spread over base of cake and refrigerate 4 hours or overnight to set.

NET CARBS 16.7G	PROTEIN 4.4G PER SERVING

 GF   VEG

SIMPLE CHEESECAKE

Serves 8 | Ready in 1 hour

600g ricotta cheese

3 large eggs

80g coconut sugar

60g brown rice flour (reserve 5 mL
for the pan)

15 mL vanilla extract

2.5 mL cinnamon

2.5 mL nutmeg

2.5 mL sea salt

45 mL grated lemon rind

60 mL fresh lemon juice

FOR SERVING:

5g cocoa powder

125g strawberries, sliced

250 mL whipping cream, whipped
(optional)

*This simple cake can be served with fresh berries, cocoa and a
dollop of whipped cream for an impressive but simple dessert.* —AT

PREHEAT the oven to 175°C (350°F). Butter the bottom of a
9-inch spring form pan, and dust it lightly with flour.

PLACE all ingredients in a food processor and blend until
smooth.

POUR the batter into spring form pan, and spread evenly.

BAKE for 50 minutes, at which point the center will feel firm
and springy to touch.

LET cool completely and then refrigerate until ready to serve.

DUST with cocoa and serve with fresh strawberries.

NET CARBS 18G	PROTEIN 11G PER SERVING

GF   VEG

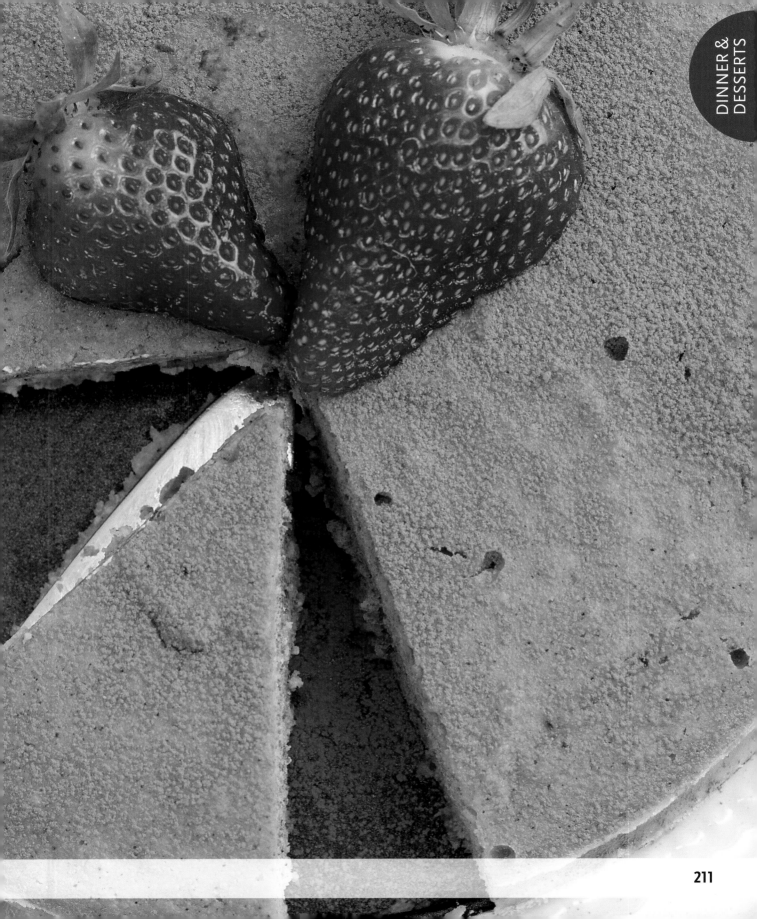

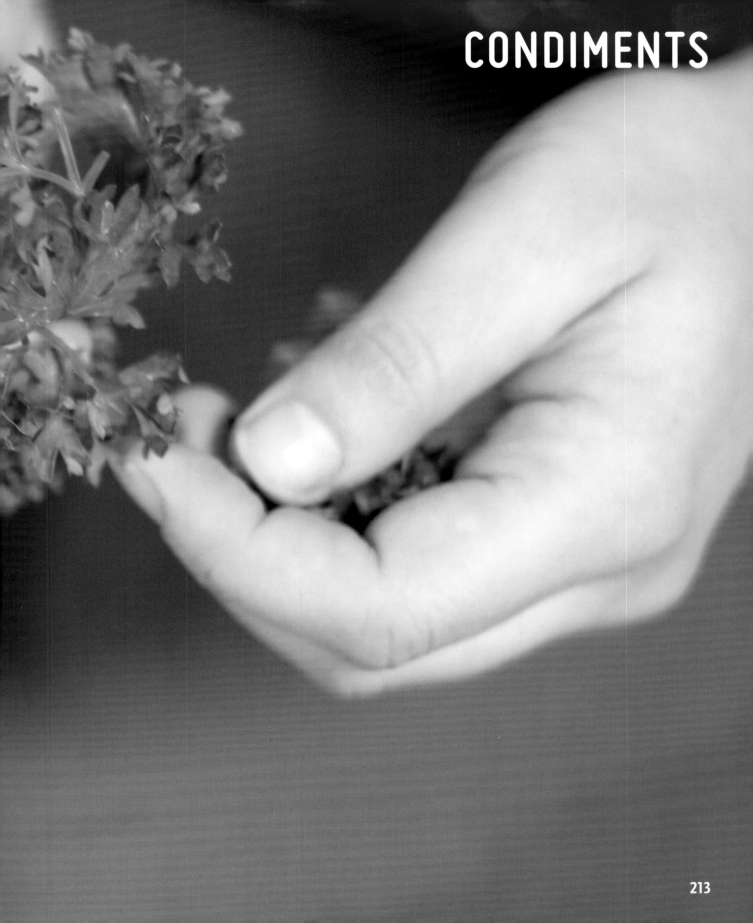

CONDIMENTS

ALPHA BALANCE™ CHILI OIL

Makes 125 mL | Ready in 1–2 days

125 mL Alpha Balance™ Oil
5 mL chili flakes

TOAST chili flakes over medium heat in a dry pan. Remove from pan and put in container. Add Alpha Balance™ Oil and steep for 1–2 days.

NET CARBS 1G FOR RECIPE

 GF VEGAN DAIRY FREE VEG

ALPHA BALANCE™ HERBS DE PROVENCE OIL

Makes 125 mL | Ready in 1–2 days

125 mL Alpha Balance™ Oil
5g shallots, minced
5 mL Herbs de Provence

PUT minced shallots and Herbs de Provence in container. Add Alpha Balance™ Oil and steep for 1–2 days.

 Once the oils are ready, they can be kept in the fridge long term, where they will solidify. The required amount can be taken out and warmed up as needed.

NET CARBS 1.8G FOR RECIPE

 GF VEGAN DAIRY FREE VEG

BARBEQUE SAUCE

Makes 1.2 L | Ready in 30 minutes

15 mL Alpha Balance™ Oil

50g onion, diced fine

9g (3 cloves) garlic, minced

341 mL (1 bottle) porter beer

10 mL vegetable bouillon

50g coconut sugar

4 allspice berries

1 clove

796 mL (1 large can) crushed tomato sauce

115g tomato paste

15 mL blackstrap molasses

15 mL ground mustard seed

30 mL apple cider vinegar

15 mL salt

15 mL hot pepper sauce

HEAT the oil in the pot over medium low. Add onions and sauté until soft. Add minced garlic and sauté until fragrant. Add the beer, bouillon and sugar, and stir until dissolved. Raise the heat and reduce to half. Grind allspice and clove, then add. Add remaining ingredients and simmer to meld flavours.

REFRIGERATE and use as required.

NET CARBS 78G	PROTEIN 13G FOR THE RECIPE

VEGAN   DAIRY FREE   VEG

BEET GINGER CHUTNEY

Makes 600 mL | Ready in 40 minutes

30 mL red palm olein

40g shallots, finely chopped

20g ginger, finely chopped

250g beets, ½ cm cubes

15g Medjool dates, minced

500 mL peppermint tea (dark)

2.5 mL cardamom

2.5 mL salt

2.5 mL apple cider vinegar

1g basil, fresh, chopped fine

15 mL Alpha Balance™ Oil

HEAT the palm olein over medium heat until it shimmers. Add the ginger and shallots. Sauté to caramelize the shallots.

ADD tea, dates, and beets, then cover and bring to a boil. Add cardamom and salt. Cook for 30 minutes until beets are tender. Take the lid off the pot, stir in the apple cider vinegar and cook off the liquid. Stir in the basil. Take off heat, stir in the Alpha Balance™ Oil, cover with lid, and let stand until serving.

STORE in airtight container in fridge for up to 2 weeks.

NET CARBS 37G	PROTEIN 5.7G FOR RECIPE

GF   VEGAN   DAIRY FREE   VEG

GURSCHE HOUSE DRESSING

Makes 500 mL | Ready in 20 minutes

125 mL lemon juice

65 mL Alpha Balance™ Oil

60 mL camelina oil

60 mL Bragg's soy seasoning

15 mL apple cider vinegar

10g garlic, minced

5g fresh oregano, chopped very fine

3g fresh thyme, leaves only, chopped fine

5g fresh sage, chopped very fine

10g fresh basil, chopped very fine

85g onion, chopped fine

1.25 mL Madras Curry Paste (optional, see page 219)

10 mL balsamic vinegar (optional)

When we make this at home we measure roughly. The amount of oil should match the lemon juice, with the Bragg's being about half of either. We use whatever herbs we have on hand, this way the dressing is never quite the same, but always tasty. It can be made in a blender, but add the chopped onions after blending to prevent them from turning bitter. – CG

COMBINE the ingredients in a 500 mL mason jar with a lid. Shake vigourously to combine. The dressing is shelf stable. If refrigerated, allow to warm to room temperature, and shake before using. The longer the dressing stands, the sweeter the onions get. Use within 2–3 weeks.

 To make a fruit vinaigrette, cut the amount of herbs in half, and add several tablespoons of fruit jam, to taste.

NET CARBS 25.3G   PROTEIN 10G FOR RECIPE

 GF   VEGAN   DAIRY FREE   VEG

HERBED FETA SOUR CREAM

Makes 185g | Ready in 20 minutes

15g fresh sweet herbs, minced
60g feta cheese
120g sour cream
Salt and pepper to taste

MIX ingredients together.

ALLOW to sit for 15 minutes to meld flavours.

 You can use whatever fresh herbs you have on hand. A mix of oregano, parsley, basil, sage, thyme and marjoram always tastes great.

NET CARBS 7.6G   PROTEIN 12.7G FOR RECIPE

 GF   VEG

HOLLANDAISE SAUCE

Makes 125 mL | Ready in 15 minutes

15 mL hot water
70g butter
2 egg yolks
2.5 mL lemon zest
5 mL lemon juice
Pinch of paprika
Dash of cayenne
Salt to taste
5g fresh basil, chopped

HEAT water until bubbles form in a shallow pot. Melt butter in small stainless steel bowl over top (as a double boiler).

ADD the yolks as the butter melts, and blend with the whip attachment of an immersion blender. Add the lemon zest, and the tablespoon of hot water. As the sauce thickens, add the lemon juice. Keep whisking constantly, about 10 minutes. When the sauce is thick, blend in the paprika, cayenne, and salt to taste.

NET CARBS 1.7G   PROTEIN 6.1G FOR THE RECIPE

 GF   VEG

THAI CURRY PASTE

Makes 250g | Ready in 30 minutes

15 mL coriander

12g peppercorns

8 mL cumin

100g green onions

30g ginger

15 mL cilantro stems

60g garlic

60 mL red palm olein

1 lime, zested (Kaffir preferred)

100g (2 stalks) lemongrass, sliced

15 mL salt

30g Thai chili peppers, membranes and seeds removed

LIGHTLY toast the coriander, peppercorns and cumin in a pan until they give off a scent. Let cool before grinding. Grind before adding to the blender. Slice green onions, lemongrass, ginger, and cilantro stems into small pieces. This will prevent the fibres from binding the blender. Cut garlic cloves into smaller chunks.

ADD lemongrass and ginger to the blender, along with the oil. Add salt, garlic, lime zest, and cilantro next. Add fresh green chili peppers. Blend until the mixture turns into a fine paste so you can't recognize individual ingredients. Salt acts as a preservative, as does the capsacin. The paste can be stored for several weeks in the fridge, or for up to a year in the freezer.

 Kaffir limes are distinct in flavour, and different than western limes. However, if you can't find kaffir limes, use a regular lime and you'll still have green curry paste. The paste can be made in the traditional manner with a mortar and pestle, or a blender. I choose the blender.

NET CARBS 28G FOR RECIPE

 GF   VEGAN   DAIRY FREE   VEG

MADRAS CURRY PASTE

Makes 250 mL | Ready in 15 minutes

30g fresh ginger

30g garlic, minced

30 mL coriander

15 mL cayenne chili powder

15 mL turmeric powder

15 mL cumin

10 mL black pepper

7.5 mL cardamom, ground

5 mL cinnamon, ground

5 mL salt

2.5 mL cloves, ground

2.5 mL nutmeg, ground

1.25 mL star anise, ground

60 mL DME™ Coconut Oil

60 mL water

5 mL apple cider vinegar

5 mL lemon juice

20 mL tamarind paste

COMBINE all ingredients and blend into a paste. May be refrigerated for several weeks, and used as required.

NET CARBS 28G	PROTEIN 6G FOR RECIPE

GF   VEGAN   DAIRY FREE   VEG

ALICIA TOBIN

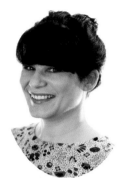

AFTER YEARS OF EATING FOOD THAT FELT WRONG, in 2006, Alicia Tobin R.H.N, discovered eating a simple, whole food diet, was the key to feeling well. In 2012 she became a Registered Holistic Nutritionist and is thrilled to help people find the foods that feel right to them. Her motto is "if it comes in a box, it isn't food anymore" and hopes that you too find the joy of being well fed, reducing stress, and finding a good night's sleep most nights. The greatest part of life is sharing good meals with good people.

Alicia lives in Vancouver where her food allergies are hardly embarrassing at all.

CHRIS GURSCHE

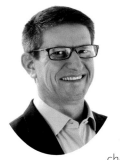

AFTER THREE MONTHS OF MARRIAGE, being sure that there were indeed more vegetables than corn, carrots and peas, I realized that if I wanted to eat as I had while living with mom, I would have to lend a hand to the cooking. And so my wife and I worked together in the kitchen, ruining cheese sauces until we learned to make them right, suffering through undercooked rice and overcooked pasta, learning along the way.

I didn't really like cooking that much, as I wanted to be adventurous, but found I was always missing an ingredient or two for the recipes I wanted to make. I was frustrated most of the time, and the meals rarely turned out the way I wanted. But I persevered.

The first breakthrough came courtesy of James Barber, *The Urban Peasant*. I watched the cooking shows because I was desperate to become a better cook. Barber said something that floored me. "If you don't have oregano, try marjoram. Or even basil. All the sweet herbs are interchangeable."

You can do that? To that point, I had been a slave to the recipe, with all the frustration that entailed. Barber opened up a world of art and creativity to me. I was liberated.

The next great step forward was when I learned the interplay of salt, sweet, and sour. That allowed me to rescue a recipe more than once, when I had added too much of a particular ingredient as I was experimenting. *Cooks Illustrated* has been a godsend: "so that's why it

works that way…" I don't approve of all their ingredients; I love their methodology.

But one of the greatest joys in the kitchen was when I discovered Molly Steven's *All About Braising*. Never have I had a cookbook so well used, where so many recipes are solid gold. Usually in a recipe book you find three, maybe five good recipes to repeat. Molly's book on braising has been the start of hundreds of family meals by now. The book's binding is unfortunately completely shot, and the recipes I have cooked again and again are now loose leaf pages. A couple of my recipes are inspired from Molly's book, and – having cooked them so often, I have modified them for a somewhat simpler style. But there is so much to appreciate in her book that I recommend you search it out and add it to your collection, if for no other reason than that most braises fit right in to the ketogenic eating style. And also, braises taste better the second day. Nobody complains about leftovers. Instead, they all want to know if there's any more of that chicken…

We find that we rarely eat out these days – what's the point when the food is so much better at home. And so I've come to the point of writing a cookbook of my own – well, half a book. Alicia has been a fantastic partner in this project, and we've spurred each other on to great tastes. Our hope is that these recipes provide a framework for your ketogenic cooking, giving you some tools for a healthier, more sustainable way of eating.

As I've adapted to ketogenesis, I find that I eat less overall. I'm still satisfied – very satisfied – eating better, feeling better, and wearing pants with a smaller waist size.

INDEX